BUTTS, GUTS, and OTHER PROBLEM AREAS

By

Jason Shea M.S., CSCS

Table of Contents

Chapter I

Nature and Nurture

Why do we store more fat in certain areas of our body versus others? An entire encyclopedia of slang terminology has developed from this "fat patterning". Saddle Bags, Bat Wings, Bingo Wings, Muffin Tops (and associated muffin top concealer, muffin top factor, Muffin Top Syndrome, the muffin tosser, a muffin tramp, and the muffin topper) Cankles, Banana Roll, Turkey Neck, Spare Tire, Beer Belly, Flags, Double Chins, Moobs, FUPA, and Pooch Belly have all been used to describe different fat patterns. But why is it that some of us develop Turkey Necks and Muffin Tops, while other develop Bat Wings and Spare Tires?

Fighting a Battle on multiple fronts

Does this situation sound familiar? Life. You know, not sleeping well for any number of reasons albeit stress, young children, working late, watching late night TV, or late night computer usage. From here we wake up tired the next morning and need a pick me up. Coffee from either Dunkin Donuts or Starbucks seems to do the trick. Oftentimes alongside the caffeine jolt comes a less than optimal food choice in the form of bagel, muffin, croissant, donut, etc.. As if this negative spiral of sleep deprivation and caffeine intake weren't causing enough damage, but then we throw in the chronic stress of daily life. What better way to alleviate this stress and calm the nerves than to indulge in a few alcoholic beverages in the evening. The negative spiral continues, and it becomes increasingly more difficult to not only stay lean, but keep additional weight from accumulating.

Physiologically speaking, what is happening here? For starters, your hormonal harmony is going haywire. Stress can lead to an increase in the storage hormone cortisol while decreasing the sensitivity of cortisol receptors throughout the body. Sleep deprivation can lead to changes in many of your hormones, further exacerbating the issue. Then, we throw a stimulant such as caffeine into the mix. In genetically susceptible individuals, caffeine can cause elevations in stress hormones while decreasing those that regulate our metabolism.

As we have heard over and over again, poor food choices can lead to dysregulation and irregularities in the management of our blood sugar, a cascade of effects on hormones, chemical burden, body fat accumulation, and more.

With all this going on, why is it our body's still insist on storing fat in specific areas while leaving other areas virtually intact? There is no definitive singular answer to this question, but rather a cascade of factors and events leading to our own individual perfect storm for fat gain. Starting from baseline, these include factors we have no "say" in including genetics, ethnicity/nationality, sex, and the environment we grew up in.

From here we are then faced with transient factors, many of which are in our control, including sleep patterns, food choices, caffeine consumption, alcohol consumption, stress levels and stress tolerance, and more. There is an infinite amount of combinations of these factors that can lead to any number of health consequences including autoimmune diseases, various illnesses, and the topic focus of this book, weight gain and problem area fat accumulation. The goal if this book is to take an objective look, based on hundreds of scientific research studies, and try to piece together some of the pieces of the problem area fat gain puzzle.

Genetics and Epigenetics

According to the Merriam-Webster dictionary, Genetics is *"scientific study of how genes control the characteristics of plants and animals"*. Our genes play a significant role in the development of our physical, mental, and even emotional health. Delving even deeper into the biological sciences is the field of study known as epigenetics. Epigenetics is loosely defined as the study of heritable changes which affect gene function without modifying the DNA sequence (2)."

Where does all this play a role in a book about problem area fat storage? It has been widely accepted that our parents have a direct physiological effect on the person we are today. A 2010 research study from *Nature* examined the effects the condition and dietary preference of grandparents, in particular the grandfather, had on the development of obesity in future generations. Two groups of male rats were fed separate diets. One group was given a healthy diet while the other was given a heavily fattening diet. Then their offspring, and their offspring's offspring were fed healthy or poor diets. The researchers found alterations in the functioning of the beta cells, cells in the pancreas that are responsible for insulin release and regulation, in the trans-generational offspring of the fattening diet group. This dysfunction led to a greater risk of obesity in the offspring.

When the offspring were then fed either poor or healthy diets, it was found that those that consumed poor diets and came from grandfathers that also consumed poor diets, were more likely to be obese than those from grandparents consuming healthy diets. Interestingly, one grandfather consuming a high fatty diet increased the risk of obesity to a greater extent than did four healthy, lean grandparent.

Not to be taken as a life sentence, the "silver lining" finding came when the researchers discovered that those offspring consuming a healthy diet, no matter what their grandparent's diet was like, were able to stay lean and healthy.

In other words, the genes were there, but the environmental dietary choices were a stronger predictor in staying lean (20)."

At the time this was one of the first studies to find a direct correlation of the role epigenetics can play on the transgenerational offspring of male subjects. How is it that twin siblings from the exact same zygote and genome can look and act nothing alike? The answer may lie in the biology sub-field known as epigenetics. The genetics may be the same, but the expression of the genome in response to environmental factors including dietary, toxin exposure, temperature, stress, and more can be dramatically altered.

In 2007 researchers discovered variants of a gene they theorized played a major role in the development of obesity. Through its impacts on satiety mechanisms in the brain, this gene, nicknamed the "fatso" gene, or FTO for short, was linked to a greater risk of obesity (7, 9, 23). That same year, a study from *Science* found that subjects carrying a single copy of this variant weighed nearly three pounds more than non-carriers, while those carrying two copies of the variant weighed nearly seven pounds more than subjects with no variants (8).

In 2010 a research team out of the Metabolism and Inflammation department at Harwell Science and Innovation Campus were able to genetically modify mice to carry two extra copies of the FTO gene. The researchers found that those mice with two extra copies of the variant actually ate more than those that did not have the extra copies. This overeating led the male mice with extra copies of the gene to be 11% heavier while the females were 22% heavier (6).

Now just because some of us may have a genetic disposition toward obesity does not mean we have a free pass to go for 2nds, 3rds, and even 4th's of the never ending pasta bowl at the Olive Garden. Or for that matter, just because there are four donuts left in the box in the office break room does not mean one person has to dutifully make sure nothing goes to waste. There is a level of personal accountability, even if the potential for obesity is genetically greater in some individuals.

Researchers have found that even if an individual is a carrier of the gene, if they choose a healthy active lifestyle, they are able to keep body fat levels in check. Named the *HELENA Study*, a research team out of the Karolinska Institute in Sweden looked at the effects one hour of physical activity would have on the attenuation of the FTO gene in the development of obesity and central body fat.

Seven hundred and fifty two students from various areas of Europe including Greece, Germany, France, Hungary, Italy, Sweden, Austria, and Spain were assessed for FTO polymorphism then monitored for physical activity. The researchers found that teenagers carrying the gene who exercised more, had lower body fat levels than those that did not participate in at least an hour of physical activity per day (22, 13).

A 2008 research study from *Diabetes* looked at the correlation between type 2 diabetes, obesity, physical activity and the presence of the FTO gene. The researchers found a significant positive correlation between type 2 diabetes and the presence of the FTO gene. Similar to the findings in the HELENA study, they also found a decreased incidence of obesity and type 2 diabetes in the FTO gene carriers who participated in regular physical activity (1). A year later, a study from *Metabolism* confirmed these findings. A positive correlation between the FTO gene, insulin, and obesity was found MONICA Study consisting of a subject pool consisting of 2769 non obese and 598 obese subjects (14).

What these studies show, is that even if you have the gene polymorphism, it does not mean you are guaranteed to become obese. An active lifestyle can dramatically curb this potential. After all, genetics plays roughly a 40-70% role in the development of obesity. Environmental, lifestyle, and personal choices account for the rest. Other studies have shown that children born to parents who are both obese can have as much as an eighty percent chance of becoming obese themselves. If one parent is obese this chance is cut in half to roughly forty percent. If neither parent is obese this chance drops below 10% (3, 4, 15, 16, 18, 27).

Studies on twins are great for determining the effects of nature vs nurture. Research out of the University of Helsinki in Finland found that genetics accounted for roughly 72% of the variance seen in male twins, while 66.4% of the variance seen in women were due to genetics. The researchers found that 27.8% and 33.6% of variance for men and women respectively, were due to non-shared environmental factors (26).

Using DXA scan, researchers analyzed regional body fat in young and older monozygotic and dizygotic twins. The researchers found that the monozygotic twins had greater similarity in body fat measures than did the dizygotic twins. Interestingly, these similarities were seen in both the young and older groups, providing further evidence that nature does play a significant role in the development of obesity (17).

A similar study followed 1974 monozygotic twins and 2097 dizygotic twins over a twenty five year period. The study found greater similarities in body type and obesity development in the monozygotic twins over that period of time (25).

A research study on Vietnam era twins out of the *American Journal of Clinical Nutrition* found that vigorous exercise played a significant role in the development of obesity in monozygotic twins. The twin that was less active showed a greater tendency toward a higher BMI while those that engaged in more exercise were often leaner. The researchers concluded that *"vigorous exercise may mitigate some of the genetic influence on obesity* (19)*."*

A separate study from the University of Helsinki looked at differences in the levels of the satiety hormone leptin and its association with obesity in twin adults aged 50-76 years old. The researchers found that 45% of the genetic variance in leptin levels in men were due to genetics, while 34% were due to genetics in women (12).

Research out of London England looked at the role genetics may play in the development of childhood obesity. Over five thousand pairs of twins between the ages of 8 and 11 had their BMI and waist circumferences measured. The researchers found that while genetics does play a significant role in the development of obesity, self-control, exercise habits, social influences and other environmental factors also play a significant role in long term weight management (5).

We have seen through the previous studies on twins that exercise can curb the genetic predisposition toward obesity.

What about diet? A 2010 thesis out of the Institute of Preventive Medicine in Denmark looked at the role diet and nutrition had on the development of obesity in twin subjects. Genetic influence was attributable to roughly 20-50% of dietary variables, especially with regards to sugar laden soft drink intake and obesity characteristics (11).

In 2002 researchers set out to determine dietary preferences in monozygotic twin subjects and compared these preferences to the prevalence of obesity in one of the twins. In each of the twenty three pairs of twins, one was lean and one was more obese. The researchers found that even though the twins grew up in the same household environment, the one that higher a greater preference toward fatty foods from young adulthood on was significantly more likely to develop obesity. The fact that one monozygotic twin was able to stay lean while the other became obese provides further evidence that our genetic pre-determination can be curbed by our dietary and lifestyle choices (21).

Interestingly though, genetics does play a significant role in weight loss in twin pairs. In 2000 a research study out of the Czech Republic found significant similarities in weight loss between identical twin subjects, but not between other twin pairs. The researchers had fourteen female twin pairs stay in a controlled supervised clinical environment for forty days while participating in a twenty eight day weight loss program followed by a five day testing period. The subjects lost an average of twenty pounds, with nearly fifteen of those pounds being lost in fat. The individual twin pair's intrapair weight loss was significantly similar, while the interpair similarities were less significant (10).

To throw a monkey wrench in the nature vs nurture debate is to look at the existing research on adopted children and body type similarities toward their genetic parents. A study out of the Danish Epidemiology Science Center looked at the obesity trends in over 3500 adoptees and compared these to the incidence of obesity in the genetic parents. The researchers found a significant correlation between the body type of the genetic parents and the adoptee, with environmental factors showing little consistency (24). A separate study from the *New England Journal of Medicine* had significantly similar findings (25).

To borrow from comedian Jeff Foxworthy, *you might be a redneck*.....You probably struggle with your weight as a result of your genetics if:

- You have been overweight since you were a young child and have difficulty losing any weight.
- The doctor strained his back while delivering you.

- In all seriousness, if both parents were/are overweight or obese your chances of developing obesity can increase up to 80%!

On the other side of the coin, environmental issues rather than genetics are to blame if:

- You are now asking yourself which chin you need to get above the bar in chin ups.
- You have switched from Under Armor to Spanx.
- You refuse to post Facebook selfies without first utilizing the "make me skinny
- Your lovehandles and bellfat begin to resemble the top of a muffin when hanging over the sides of your skinny jeans.
- People begin asking you how far along you are
- The drive thru operator at Taco Bell knows you on a first name basis.

In the next chapter let's delve a little deeper into the topic of fat.

Chapter II

Finishing the Frusen Gladje

Grasso gordo gruby gras

Have you ever wondered how exactly does that fast food hamburger, side order of French fries, Strawberry milkshake, and apple pie served in cardboard cutout make us fat? Physiologically speaking, what actions go on inside our body after we have eaten the last spoonful of Frusen Gladja that so readily plasters deposits of unsightly fat around our midsection or on our thighs. In other words, how does what we put in our mouth turn to the fat on our buns, above our hips, below our chins, and around our bellies?

From 1971 to 2000 the average caloric consumption of women has increased by 335 calories per day. The average man has increased his calories by 168 calories per day. According to a 2010 WebMD blog post *"the average American woman is 5'4", has a waist size of 34-35" and weighs between 140-150lbs with a dress size of 12-14. Fifty years ago, the average woman was 5'3 with a waist size of approximately 24-25", she weighed about 120lbs and wore an 8 for a waist size (32)"*

The term fat, derived from the Latin word *obesus*, was used to describe individuals whose health was suffering due to overindulgence. Fat refers to fat cells known as adipocytes, that are stored in different areas throughout our body. There are three main categories of fat found in the human body: visceral fat, subcutaneous fat, and brown adipose tissue (BAT). Each of these serves a different function in the body.

Fat is primarily stored in designated fat storage cells called adipocytes. Adipocytes are stored in different areas throughout the body, primarily under the skin or in regions surrounding vital organs (for protection) called visceral fat. Most of the fat inside the adipocytes is in the form of a triacylglycerol *(TAG or triglyceride).* Triacylglycerol are composed of a backbone (glycerol) with 3 fatty acid tails.

In several research studies, fat tissue has been found to be an endocrine tissue. Researchers have identified nearly eighty different proteins that are secreted by fat cells (35). Some of the major hormones secreted by fat tissue include leptin, resistin, and estrogen, each of which can play an active role in the development of obesity.

Leptin is a satiety hormone that signals the brain to let us know when we are full. Resistin is a pro-inflammatory hormone that has been shown to play a role in insulin resistance, while estrogen has been associated with various diseases including cancers, Parkinson's Disease, and obesity.

Studies have shown that obese adults and children do not necessarily eat more than their lean counterparts, rather they expend less calories, which in turns leads to slower metabolic rates. Researchers found that lean individuals were more efficient at regulating energy intake associated with active and inactive periods (15).

Fat cells also secrete signaling proteins known as cytokines. These play an important role in the body's response to inflammation, infection, and other disease. A major cytokine released from the adipose tissue is *Tumor Necrosis Factor-alpha*, or TNF-a. Based on research from the mid 1970's, TNF-a was named for its ability to cause death of toxin induced tumors in mice (10).

Why is that important? Because cancer, Alzheimer's disease, and other diseases associated with inflammation have been linked to dysfunctions in the production and regulation of *Tumor Necrosis Factor-alpha*. TNF-a also plays a role in obesity as it is associated with appetite suppression, insulin regulation, and the stimulation of the release of cortisol through its actions on corticotropin releasing hormone.

Types of Fat

Brown Adipose Tissue

Metabolically active type of fat that is responsible for thermoregulation as it turns food into heat. Has more capillaries than white fat. High mitochondrial content gives BAT it's brown coloration.

Neutral Colored Adipose Tissue (*brite*)

White fat tissue that expresses thermogenic capacity.

White Subcutaneous Fat

Most common type of fat in the body, this metabolically inactive fat directly under the skin, found about the hips, thighs, belly, and butt (*think cellulite*). Subcutaneous fat produces the hormone adiponectin, a hormone that plays an important role in glucose regulation and lipid metabolism in insulin sensitive tissues. The larger the fat cells, the less adiponectin you produce, potentially leading to metabolic disorders. The smaller the fat cells, the more adiponectin produced.

White Visceral Fat

The deep fat that surrounds our internal organs, visceral fat releases immune system substances called cytokines that can affect insulin production and promote chronic inflammation. Visceral fat also plays a role in the development of cholesterol as it empties toxins, metabolites, and fatty acids into the bloodstream and liver (19). Chronic visceral inflammation is seen in the development of abdominal obesity.

Did you know that visceral fat is more metabolically active than subcutaneous fat? It is also more sensitive to the effects of cortisol due to its higher content of cortisol receptors. Did you also know that digestive health and intestinal issues, in particular the small intestine, can promote fat accumulation about the abdomen because of where the small intestine in positioned in the body (5)?

Cellulite

Cellulite is the uneven, dimpled/marbled looking fat that often rears its head about the butt, thighs, and midsection. It has been referred to as appearing like cottage cheese or an orange peel.

Our fat cells are stored in compartments just below the dermis. This layer of subcutaneous fat is just above a layer of connective tissue that is housed between the fat and muscle tissue.

When the stability of the connective collagen tissue layer is weakened due to a multitude of reasons including hormonal changes, poor circulation, lack of exercise, hydration issues, smoking, poor nutrition, age, gender, estrogenic toxins, and metabolic changes, hard fibrous bands may form in the connective tissue. The subcutaneous fat is then compressed, leading to herniation. This is when the "cottage cheese/orange peel" appearance presents (36).

There are gender differences in this collagen tissue that increase the risk of cellulite appearance. Men may have a thicker dermis layer that increases the risk of internal expansion, while women run the risk of external expansion leading to an increased risk of cellulite appearance (34). The good news is that females who lose weight seem to make the appearance of cellulite disappear.

> In a 2001 study out of Munich, Germany, scientists treated Holsteins with two common feedlot growth promoters: trenbolone acetate and melengestrol acetate. Then, over the next two months, the researchers analyzed all of the animal's manure, nearly 100 tons of it. The researchers found that roughly 10% of both the trenbolone and melengestrol was passed into the feces. Of particular concern were the scientists finding regarding the length of time the steroids survived in the manure. **The researchers found the drugs were able to resist bacterial breakdown for up to 260 days**, unless spread throughout the fields, which they found dramatically shortened the half-life. At the end of the study the researchers questioned "what share of the drugs' disappearance might be the result of runoff-versus microbial breakdown- remains an open question." (38)

This process of cellulite appearance occurs in four phases:

1. Changes in microcirculation.

2. Fluids are released and trapped in the extracellular space.
3. Fibrous bands begin to form in the connective tissue, adipose tissues increase in size, and dimpling begins to appear.
4. Bands thicken and harden, leading to herniation of subcutaneous fat.

Other factors that may affect the development of cellulite include:

- Genetics
- Gender
- Age
- Hormones (estrogen, thyroid, insulin, prolactin, and epinephrine/norepinephrine
- Race
- Obesity (the more fat you have, the more pressure on the connective tissue to herniate)
- Alcohol consumption
- Circulatory health
- Smoking
- Stress

Fat Adapted

The hormone insulin and the catecholamines play a significant role in fat cell mobilization. When insulin levels are low and epinephrine levels are elevated, stored fat can be broken down into separate fatty acids and glycerol. These are then mobilized into the bloodstream. In the bloodstream, the fatty acids can bind to the carrier protein albumin, which aids in shuttling the fatty acids to the muscles, either to be used as fuel or stored as fat.

> **Did you know?** In 1988, the EU banned importation of meats that came from hormone treated animals. Walk into any grocery store around the EU and look at the labeling of the meats. (41)

For these fatty acids to cross from the bloodstream into the cell, more carrier proteins are required. According to a 2008 study out of the *Department of Human Health and Nutritional Sciences* at the University of Guelph, the protein FAT/CD36, short for fatty acid translocase, regulates this transport into the mitochondria during exercise (23).

> **Acetyl -L- Carnitine** is a highly researched dietary supplement that has been found to improve fat loss and fatty acid utilization. The substrate carnitine acts as a fatty acid transporter, shuttling these fat cells into the mitochondria to be stored or used as fuel.

The enzyme CPT1, (Carnitine Palmitoyltransferase), also plays a role in the burning of long chain fatty acids in the mitochondria. FATP, (fatty acid transport protein), and FABPpm, (fatty acid binding protein), also plays a role in the utilization of fatty acids by the mitochondria (7).

Depending on factors including food intake, physical activity, and hormonal status, the fatty acids may be stored or burned as fuel.

Fat can be burned during exercise, post exercise, and at rest. If your body has become *"fat adapted"*, you will be much more efficient at utilizing fat as a fuel source at various workout intensity levels, especially during longer duration workouts. There are three specific energy systems utilized during activity:

1. **ATP/Phosphate Energy System:** This is the high intensity short duration energy system, ranging from roughly 0 to 20s of all out work.
2. **Glycolytic Energy System:** Depending on the individual this can range from 20 to 90s of high to moderate intensity.
3. **Aerobic/Oxidative Energy System:** Dependent upon a trainee's efficiency at utilizing fat as a fuel source, this can range from 120s and up.

These systems are not absolutes, as oftentimes, your body will require a mixed usage of these systems for energy. Individual factors including genetics, dietary macronutrient intake, muscle fiber content, training status, and more can impact these energy systems.

It has often been thought that, depending upon the trainee's efficiency at utilizing fat as a fuel source, fat burning occurs at roughly 60% intensity oxidative/aerobic work. It should be recognized that this is dependent on more than just the intensity of the exercise. Body fat %, genetics, muscle mass, diet, macronutrient intake prior to workout, caffeine, hydration status, and more can all play a role in fat burning.

Another great fat burning benefit to exercise, especially at higher intensities, is the elevated energy expenditure post workout, otherwise known as EPOC. EPOC stands for Excess Post Exercise Oxygen Consumption. A 2012

> Mitochondria density (the # of mitochondria per unit of muscle) is lower in obese individuals. This may play a significant role in the decreased ability for obese individuals to use fat as a fuel source.

study from the *Journal of Translational Medicine* looked at the post workout resting energy expenditure in seventeen subjects after bouts of high intensity interval training and more traditional resistance training. The researchers found a significant increase in resting energy expenditure twenty-two hours after the workout in the group that performed the high intensity protocols versus the traditional training group (31).

A separate study, this one from the exercise physiology lab at Purdue University, also looked at different exercise intensities, but also took into account the duration of EPOC. On separate occasions, the researchers had 10 triathletes perform:

- short duration high intensity workout,
- short duration low intensity workout,
- and long duration low intensity workout

on a cycle ergometer. The researchers found similar EPOC durations from the short duration high intensity workout and the long duration low intensity workout. Of particular significance was the caloric expenditure during this time period. The high intensity workouts yielded over two times greater caloric expenditure post-exercise than did the low intensity workouts no matter the duration (39).

A 2014 study from the *European Journal of Applied Physiology* measured the magnitude and duration of EPOC as well as heart rate recovery from twenty minute bouts of running at 60%, 70%, and 80% VO2max. The researchers found significant differences in the magnitude of EPOC with each exercise intensity. They concluded it was the magnitude of EPOC that had a greater metabolic effect than duration of EPOC (28).

Studies have shown that for the same energy expenditure during a workout, lower body workouts result in a significantly greater magnitude and duration of EPOC when compared to upper body exercise (27).

We have seen that EPOC is significantly affected by greater intensities of training, especially in lower body exercise. Studies have also shown that the type of exercise, more specifically strength training can have a significant effect on EPOC. When we workout, we are in essence breaking down muscle tissue on a micro level. Associated with this breakdown is the work required by the body to rebuild this muscle back baseline, then further work is required for nervous system/musculoskeletal system adaptation and growth.

A 2014 study looked at the effect the type...or, ahem.....the name of the workout had on a trainee's appetite post workout. The researchers had nearly one hundred subjects participate in the same twenty-minute cycle ergometer workout at roughly 55-65% VO2max. The only difference was that the researchers altered the names of the workout, with half the group doing the "endurance" workout and the other half performing the "fat burning" workout. Of significance, the exercisers who participated in the workout under the "fat burning" designation were more likely to indulge in larger quantities of food than those performing the same exact workout, only named differently (18).

Do different intensity weight training workloads have different effects on EPOC? A group of 14 female subjects were taken through two separate workouts and then had their blood lactate levels, oxygen consumption, respiration, and heart rate measured directly after the workout and 20, 60, and 120 minutes afterward. The first workout consisted of nine separate exercises for two sets of 15 reps at 45% of the subjects 8RM, while the second workout consisted of the same nine exercises with two sets of 8 repetitions at 85% of the subjects 8RM. **The researchers found the resulting EPOC to be significantly greater, in fact, nearly double, when the subjects performed the heavy resistance low repetition workout** (42).

Quite possibly, an even greater level of EPOC may exist with intensive circuit training. A 1999 research study looked at the effects 20 or 60 second rest periods during a 20 rep circuit had on post workout oxygen consumption. **The EPOC was nearly 25% greater one-hour post workout when the shorter rest intervals were incorporated**. The shorter rest intervals also led to a greater caloric expenditure at one-hour post workout, while the longer rest period led to a greater overall total energy expenditure (22).

A 1997 study from *Medicine and Science in Sports and Exercise* had twenty-six female subjects break down into three separate groups: no exercise, 1-2 thirty-minute cardio workouts per week, or 3-4 thirty-minute cardio workouts per week. The researchers that the subcutaneous fat mass was significantly decreased with training 3-4 times per week, while the visceral fat was more affected by a caloric deficit, either via greater energy expenditure or less calories consumed (1).

An interesting study from the 2011 *Journal of Strength and Conditioning Research* looked at the effects 60 and 180 second rest intervals had on either large or smaller muscle groups. Subjects performed either leg press or chest flys for 5 sets of 10 reps each at the subjects 15RM for each exercise. The leg press induced greater oxygen consumption than the chest fly at both rest intervals, while there was significantly elevated EPOC in the leg press sets with one-minute rest intervals. In essence, this study shows that the larger the muscle mass worked, combined with shorter rest intervals, the greater the oxygen consumption and energy expenditure during and post workout (17).

Does the order of the exercise affect EPOC? A research team out of the Research Facility in Physical Activity at the University of Porto in Portugal looked at the effect the order of resistance and aerobic exercise during a workout had on post workout oxygen consumption. The researchers had the subjects perform one workout that consisted of 30 minutes at 80-85% on the treadmill followed by strength training that consisted of five exercises at three sets of 10 reps. The order was then switched for a second workout.

The researchers were unable to find significant differences in one hour EPOC, though they did find higher respiratory exchange ratio and significantly greater volume of carbon dioxide expiration in the strength followed by aerobic training group (30).

Although EPOC does not differ significantly with regards to order of the exercise, it may be more beneficial to perform the strength work first, followed by cardiovascular or interval training. As seen in the previously mentioned research study, there is a greater respiration exchange ratio and higher volume of carbon dioxide exhalation associated with this order of training. Strength and hypertrophy results may also be greater when utilizing this intra-session exercise order. Common sense tells us that training for strength while in a fatigued state may not be optimal. For example, finding one's three rep max deadlift after a three-mile run may not be the most effective method for strength testing, nor can it be recommended as the safest.

Strength training while energy substrate levels are adequate has been shown in research to be more effective with regards to gains in strength. A 2012 study from *Experimental Gerontology* looked the strength and hypertrophy results in the quadriceps musculature in subjects performing workouts three times per week consisting of strength followed by cardio or vice versa.

While both groups experienced similar gains in conditioning and hypertrophy, the intra-session strength training followed by endurance work yielded significantly greater results in strength (8). A 2013 study from *Age* had similar findings (9).

A more recent study from the *International Journal of Sports Medicine* also found that after twelve weeks of two times per week of strength training followed by aerobic training elicited significantly greater lower body strength and hypertrophy results (33).

Looking at the order of resistance and cardio exercise from a hormonal perspective, a group of researchers from the Human and Environmental Physiology research unit at the University of Ottawa had type 1 diabetic subjects perform workouts consisting of 45 minutes of weight training followed by 45 minutes of cardio or vice versa. They found lower glucose levels after the cardio section of the workout no matter the exercise order. The researchers did find that **performing cardio after the resistance training was more advantageous to the stability of blood sugar levels than cardio before resistance** (44).

> ****Side Note:** *in personal interview with world renowned Cardiovascular and Hypertension specialist, Dr. Mark Houston, he has suggested that for improving cardiovascular health, the optimal method and order of exercise during a workout to be intensive strength training for roughly 40 minutes followed by 20 minutes of intense interval conditioning.*

Are there other ways can manipulate EPOC?

Caffeine

➤ A group of researchers out of Cal State University gave strength trained subjects either 6mg/kg of caffeine or a placebo and had them complete an intense strength training workout at 70-80% 1RM of an exercise. The researchers found that there was little difference in calories burned during the workout, even though there was roughly a **15% difference in oxygen consumption and energy expenditure in the group that ingested caffeine prior to the workout** (4).

Antagonistic Muscle Group Super Setting

➤ Another method of increasing the energy expenditure of the workout is to include antagonistic muscle group super sets. A 2010 study from the *Journal of Strength and Conditioning Research* had healthy and active subjects participate in antagonistic muscle group superset training and traditional straight set training and compared EPOC in both training protocols. With one week of recovery between each workout variation, the researchers found the **one-hour post workout EPOC to be on average 25% greater from the antagonistic superset workout than the traditional straight sets workout**. Another significant outcome was the differences in time dependent energy expenditure. Relative to time, **the superset workout resulted in 25% greater energy expenditure** as expressed in kj/min than did the traditional straight sets workout (26).

Green Tea

➢ Green tea, or the catechins in green tea, have also been shown to increase energy expenditure and fat burning over a 24-hour period. Subjects were given either a green tea extract consisting of 90mg EGCG and 50mg of caffeine, 50mg of caffeine, or a placebo 3 times daily at meals. **The group that ingested the green tea extract consisting of both caffeine and catechins had the largest increase in 24-hour energy expenditure and fat oxidation** while the effects of the caffeine ingestion were minimal. What this study shows is that it may be other compounds besides the caffeine in green tea that induce increase in energy expenditure and associated fat burning (14).

Spicy Foods (red peppers)

➢ Spicy food may also be an effective agent in speeding up one's metabolic rate. Research from the *British Journal of Nutrition* looked at the effects spicy food, in particular red peppers, had on energy expenditure in two groups ingesting two different types of diets. The subjects were given a breakfast consisting of either high fat, high fat with the red pepper, high carb, or high carb with red pepper. **The high fat meal combined with the red pepper yielded the highest rate of fat oxidation and diet induced thermogenesis** while the high carb meal without the pepper yielded the lowest rate of fat burning. The researchers concluded that the addition of the red pepper greatly increased both fat burning and diet induced thermogenesis (45).

MCT's (Medium Chain Triglycerides)

➢ A 1996 double-blind, randomized study looked at the effects medium chain triglycerides could have on energy expenditure. Through the use of a respiratory chamber, researchers were able to determine the effects 10g of medium chain or long chain triglycerides three times per day had on 24-hour energy expenditure. <u>The researchers found roughly a 5% increase in energy expenditure per day with the consumption of 30g of medium chain triglycerides per day</u> (13).

➢ A separate study from the *Canadian Journal of Physiology and Pharmacology* looked at the effects one week of medium chain triglyceride intake had on a zone type of diet, with 40% of the calories coming from fat, 45% from carbs, and 15% from protein. Subjects either had roughly 60% or 1% of their total fat ingested in the form of medium chain triglycerides. Though the researchers did not find significant differences in total energy expenditure, they did find significant elevations in fat oxidation with higher medium chain triglyceride intake (2).

EGCG

➤ There is also some positive research on different antioxidants that can an effect on metabolism and energy expenditure. **EGCG, the one of the major antioxidants in green tea and resveratrol, a major antioxidant found in red and white wines, have both been shown to increase metabolism and energy expenditure** (29).

Polyphenols

➤ The antioxidants in coffee, known as polyphenols, have been shown in placebo controlled, double-blind, crossover studies to enhance fat oxidation. A 2013 study had 9 male subjects consume 329 mg of coffee polyphenols every day for four weeks. The researchers compared their energy expenditure and fat utilization to 9 other male subjects consuming the placebo beverage. **Increases in energy expenditure and fat oxidation were found in the coffee polyphenol group only** (40).

➢ Combining different metabolism enhancing agents can also increase thermogenesis. A 2013 study from the *European Journal of Nutrition* found that **subjects could increase their diet induced thermogenesis by roughly 50% with the ingestion of both chili and medium chain triglycerides** (11).

A few interesting points about Exercise and Fat Metabolism:

- Exercise can increase the shuttling of fatty acids into powerhouse (mitochondria) of muscle cells.
- Training can lead to increases in capillary amount which can lead to more fat being shuttled to the muscle.
- Trained subjects are more adept at using more fat as fuel than non-trained/untrained subjects (25)

There are also certain compounds that can decrease energy expenditure and fat oxidation. One such compound is the simple sugar, Fructose. A 2012 study out of the *European Journal of Clinical* Nutrition looked at the effects 10 weeks of glucose or fructose ingestion had on energy expenditure and energy substrate utilization. The fructose ingestion group had significant decreases in resting energy expenditure and fat oxidation while showed a significant increase in carbohydrate oxidation (12)

XX, XY's and low hanging fruit

A 2011 study from *Diabetes* found that women stored more fatty acids in their subcutaneous fat areas than men. The researchers also found men had a tendency to store fat more in the upper body while women stored more in the lower body (3).

Men were found to have larger visceral fat cells while women were found to have larger gluteal fat cells (6). Women may have greater ability to burn carbs, while men may be more efficient at burning fat (6).

Hormones play a role as well. Testosterone has been shown to have an impact on fatty acid oxidation as well. A 2012 study from *PloS One* found that subjects with healthy testosterone levels oxidized more fatty acids over a six-hour period than did those subjects with low testosterone levels. The researchers also found that the men with lower testosterone stored more fatty acids in the subcutaneous fat depots of the lower body than men with healthy testosterone (37).

The proportion of fatty acids stored in lower body subcutaneous adipose tissue were greater in men with low testosterone versus those men with normal testosterone.

Estrogen also plays a role in this. Researchers have found that women going through menopause often lose fat around their subcutaneous fat areas of the thighs and buttocks, while gaining more fat about the abdominal region (24, 21, 20, 43). Studies have also shown that when postmenopausal women undergo hormone replacement therapy, they begin to decrease fat accumulation about the midsection while gaining more fat about the thighs and buttocks (21).

A 1999 study on male to female transsexuals found that when the men were given estrogen it altered their fat distribution patterning. They began to shift from storing fat in the abdominal region to storing fat about the thighs and buttocks (16).

More on how our hormones can affect where we store our body fat in the next chapter.......

Chapter III

Hormones, Skinfolds and Where You Store Fat

Did you know that your hormones play a critical role in where you are storing your body fat? The late research scientist Per Bjorntorp is quite possibly the most significant contributor to the science of hormonal control and regulation of body fat storage.

In some of his earlier works, Bjorntorp was already beginning to correlate fat distribution patterns and their hormonal regulation. Noticing deficiencies in certain anabolic hormones or excess secretion of storage and/or catabolic hormones led to fat distribution patterns in men and women. From his early research on serum androgen levels and fat distribution in women to his studies on testosterone replacement in men with excess belly fat, Bjorntorp's work has played a critical role in the science of hormones and fat distribution.

Truly a pioneer in this field, Bjorntorp began seeing similarities in fat distribution patterning and hormonal profiles of his subjects as early as the late 80's early 90's. In 1991, the *International Journal of Obesity* printed his research paper **"Adipose tissue distribution and function",** in which Bjorntorp provided some magnificent insight into the hormonal regulation of fat storage. Excesses or deficiencies in certain hormones could lead to fat accumulation in different areas of the human body.

Many of Bjorntorp's other works were published in the pages of other highly respected journals, from the aptly named *"Hormonal control of regional fat destruction (1997)"* found in the pages of the *Human Reproduction* publication, to his works in *Hormonal Research* and the *International Journal of Obesity* including *"Endocrine-metabolic pattern and adipose tissue distribution (1993)", "Adipose tissue distribution and function (1991)",* and *"The regulation of adipose tissue distribution in humans (1996*)", Bjorntorp's work was truly cutting edge.

How do some of your major hormones affect weight gain? If highly insulinogenic chemical laden processed foods make up the majority of your diet, the hormone insulin may be compromised. More may be required, leading to a decrease in its action, efficiency, and sensitivity. If you are stressed, whether physically (poor nutrition is stressful on the body) or emotionally, your body may increase the production of the stress hormone cortisol, which signals the body to go into storage mode. Storage of calories and eventually fat accumulation may result.

If your thyroid is not functioning optimally, your metabolism may slow down, which in turn may lead to weight gain. If your testosterone levels are similar to those seen in pygmy goats, you may see a dramatic in increase in body fat accumulation due to the decreases in lean muscle tissue. With a decrease in testosterone, you may see an increase in the *"female"* hormone estrogen, which is conveniently stored in fat cells. With more estrogen, you will need more and larger fat cells to accommodate.

Growth hormone has an effect on fat loss through its actions on lipolysis. GH can stimulate the receptors on fat cells to increase mobilization, so they can be used as fuel.

Through stimulatory hormones, the pituitary gland is responsible for the regulation of the production of many of the major hormones including growth hormone, androgens, thyroid, estrogen, and cortisol. For instance, the pituitary gland produces luteinizing hormone and follicle stimulating hormone which in turn stimulate the production of testosterone in the testes.

Adrenocorticotrophic hormone is another hormone produced in the pituitary. ACTH stimulates the adrenal gland to produce cortisol and DHEA. The same goes for the pituitary's role in thyroid hormone production, with thyroid stimulating hormone being produced in this "master gland".

Other hormones such as insulin, the catecholamines, glucagon, serotonin, and neuropeptide Y are under the regulation of other glands such as the adrenals and brain. Fat cells have even been shown to be endocrine tissue themselves, with the production of hormones such as leptin and ghrelin.

Not only do many of the hormones stimulate the release and regulation of other hormones and the accompanying bodily processes, but they are also a part of a negative feedback loop which in turn inhibits the release of certain hormones. Basically, the hormonal system is one large feedback loop, in which a hormone stimulates the release of another hormone from an organ. The release of that hormone will then cause the desired/undesired physical response, leading the release of yet another hormone which then plays an inhibitory role to the actions of the stimulatory hormones.

Apples and Pears

A study published in *The Journal of American Medical Association* looked at how people of different body fat distribution patterns, apple or pear, respond to different types of diets. The goal was to use two different diets that affected insulin sensitivity and see how these diets performed in subjects with different fat distribution patterns. The diets were low carb and low fat. Understanding that the apple fat distribution pattern subjects secrete more insulin post meal and that the pears secreted less. The apples lost more weight on the low carb diet and were able to maintain for 18 months, while the pears lost weight on both diets as long as they had a reduced caloric intake.

The downside of being a pear was that the weight came off more slowly and was also gained more quickly (6).

Did you know that where you store your fat has been linked to cardiovascular disease risk factors?

A 1989 study from *The American Journal of Clinical Nutrition* found both the ratio of triceps and subscapular skinfold measurements and waist to hip girths were associated with higher concentrations of serum triglycerides and lower levels of good HDL cholesterol (11).

In keeping with the CVD risk factors and body fat storage patterns a separate, much earlier study from *The American Journal of Clinical Nutrition,* looked at the reliability of the triceps skinfold thickness versus the subscapular skinfold thickness as a measure of overall obesity.

The researchers found that in obese women, the triceps skinfold measurement was greater than the subscapular measurement in 83% of those women tested. The subscapular measurement was greater in only 12% of the subjects. The researchers stated *"We were struck by the fact that in a number of particularly obese women there was a notable absence of a marked excess of fat in the region of the back (subscapular) while at the same time in all instances the thickness of the triceps skin fold indicated marked excessive adipose tissue. Thus, there appear to be obese women who have excessive fat deposits on the upper arm but not on the back (26)."*

Another earlier study from *The American Journal of Clinical Nutrition* looked at the relationships between skinfold thickness and blood sugar/blood fats in normal men. The researchers found the *"highest triglyceride levels were found in men who were moderately obese and had acquired their excess adiposity during adult life. The thickness of the scapular and costal skinfolds was strongly correlated with the other measures of fatness (1)."*

An interesting finding of the study was the correlation between forearm thickness and metabolic disorders, in particular high serum triglycerides. The researchers expressed *"**It is apparent that the thinner the forearm, the more strongly is central adiposity correlated with serum triglyceride concentration.** The man whose innate state of thinness is indicated by a thin forearm could thus become obese only at the cost of overloading his existing centrally located adipose cells, while the naturally obese man, generously endowed with adipose cells, could easily expand his adipose tissue without overloading any one cell. The fact that the mean triglyceride levels in the innately thin man who becomes obese are higher than in the* innately obese man suggests that hyperglyceridemia may result from overloading of existing adipose cells. This hypothesis would account for the frequently normal triglyceride concentrations in very obese men and the high triglyceride concentrations in thin men who have gained even a modest amount of weight (1)."

"The correlation between weight gain during adult life and fat thickness of the trunk but not of the extremities lends some support to the hypothesis that there are two types of obesity: 1) hereditary obesity, or obesity acquired very early in life, in which adiposity is generalized and involves the extremities as

> **Where is Wim Hoff when you need him?**
>
> "Some years ago, Scholander proposed a series of studies of thermal and metabolic responses to moderate cold exposure in primitive people suspected of experiencing frequent and prolonged cold exposure. Subjects slept or tried to sleep in 0-5 degree C in a single thickness sleeping bag. Skinfolds were measured at 10 sites: cheek, chin, upper arm, subscapular, side abdomen, iliac crest, knee and calf. Even though they had lower body fat than the Caucasian controls, Peruvian Quechua Indians from high altitudes and Lapps had low rectal temperatures and maintained high extremity temperatures suggesting a redistribution of body heat. Acclimatized Norwegian students reacted somewhat like the Alacaluf and Eskimo with high metabolic rates and warm extremities (7)."

well as the trunk; and 2) acquired, or perhaps cultural obesity resulting from overeating and underactivity after maturity in which obesity is largely of the trunk and not extremities (1)."

The researchers concluded *"that there are two kinds of fat men: those with thin forearms who are by nature thin but who have gained weight during adult life, and those with fat forearms who have been fat all their lives. Abdominal skinfold thickness greater than 20mm is associated with serum triglyceride levels that are markedly higher in naturally thin men than naturally fat men (1)."*

Gender Differences in Fat Patterning

A 2005 study (3) found that a gender difference exists in the actual skinfolds themselves. The researchers found that females actually have….ahem….thinner skin than males (thank you science) with identical skinfold measurements. These identical measurements actually contained different concentrations of fat compared to their male counterparts (3).

Impact of Heritage/Ethnicity on Fat Patterning

A 2011 study from *Medicine and Science in Sports and Exercise* looked at body fat patterning in different ethnic groups. The researchers found those of Hispanic descent to have the highest skinfold thickness across the four sites for women, while the findings were similar in men (4). The following are graphs of their findings:

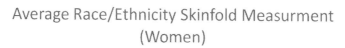

Average Race/Ethnicity Skinfold Measurment (Women)

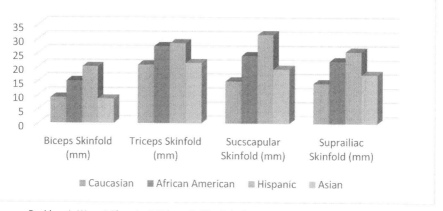

Davidson L, Wang J, ThorntonJ, Kaleem Z, Silva-Palacios F, Pierson R, Heymsfield S, Gallagher D. **Predicting fat percent by skinfolds in Racial Groups: Durnin and Womersley Revisited.** *Medicine and Science in Sports and Exercise.* 43(3); Pp 542-549. 2011.

Average Race/Ethnicity Skinfold (Men)

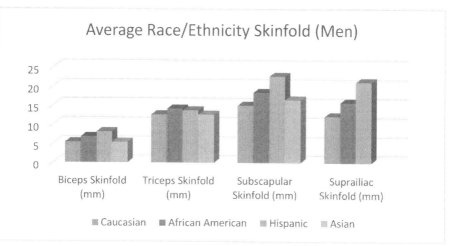

Davidson L, Wang J, ThorntonJ, Kaleem Z, Silva-Palacios F, Pierson R, Heymsfield S, Gallagher D. **Predicting fat percent by skinfolds in Racial Groups: Durnin and Womersley Revisited.** *Medicine and Science in Sports and Exercise.* 43(3); Pp 542-549. 2011.

An earlier study from the *Annals of New York Academy of Sciences* looked at the ethnic differences for 10 skinfold sites (7). The findings are below

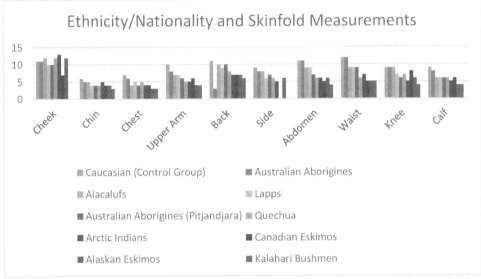

Eisner R. **Skinfold thickness in primitive peoples native to cold climates**. *Annals of New York Academy of Sciences.* 110; Pp 503-514. 1963.

Impact of Training on Fat Patterning?

Can the type of training you do affect where you lose fat from? In a 2005 study from *The British Journal of Sports Medicine*, researchers followed 24 male and 13 female runners who engaged in intense training over a three-year period. The runners were classified into groups according to their best performance capabilities according to event; sprint trained consisted of 100m and 400m; endurance trained consisted of 800m, 1500m, 3000, 5000m, 10,000m, and marathon.

To be included in this study, athletes were required to compete at a national or international level for at least two years. 12 of the males and 8 of the females were Olympic athletes. All athletes trained six or seven days a week (20-25hrs) during the season.

Skinfold thicknesses were taken at the biceps, triceps, subscapular, pectoral, iliac crest, abdominal, front thigh, and medial calf. After one, two, and three years of training, there was a significant increase in performance and decreases in the sum of six skinfolds. There were no significant differences in body weight, triceps, subscapular, pectoral, and iliac crest skinfolds (9).

The researchers found that 30 runners had significantly increased their performance, while decreasing the sum of six skinfolds. These 30 athletes also saw statistically significant drops in abdominal, front thigh and medial calf skinfolds after three years of training. The researchers also found that 7 runners had actually decreased their performance, while increasing the sum of six skinfolds (9).

In the sprinters, the changes in performance were associated with the changes in front thigh and medial calf skinfolds as well as the sum of six skinfolds.

The researchers concluded that their results suggest that the loss of body fat is specific to muscular groups used in sprint and endurance trained athletes (9).

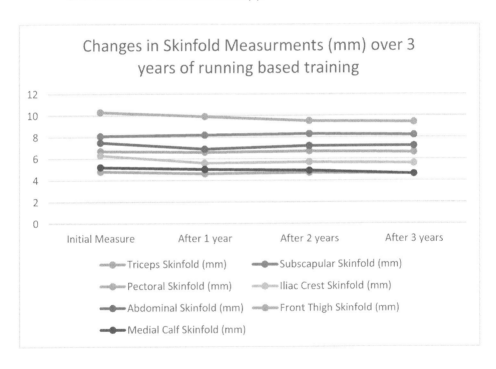

Changes in Skinfold Measurments (mm) over 3 years of running based training

Are skinfold measurements and predictor equations accurate depicters of total body adiposity?

In 2012, a research team in Brussels, Belgium analyzed the correlations between the actual caliper skinfold measurements using three different equations and the results of the DEXA scan body fat analysis in 128 subjects. The researchers measured 14 skinfold sites:

- Triceps
- Subscapular
- Scapular (oblique fold at inferior angle of scapula)
- Biceps
- Forearm 1 (vertical fold at maximum girth lateral aspect, hand supinated)
- Forearm 2 (vertical fold at maximum girth anterior aspect, hand supinated)
- Iliac Crest horizontal
- Iliac Crest Vertical
- Chest
- Supraspinalis
- Abdominal
- Front Thigh
- Thigh
- Medial Calf

5 out of 6 of the best predictor sites were on the lower limbs, with the front thigh, rear thigh, medial calf, and supra spinal being the best. The authors noted that the triceps site, which is a commonly used skinfold site in predictor equations, ranked eleventh

An unexpected finding is the high correlation for lower limb sites. Of the six best sites, all but one was on the lower limbs. The triceps, a highly favored site for "fat" prediction and considered to be the single indicator adipose tissue ranked a poor eleventh. The best predictors were front thigh, medial calf, rear thigh and supra spinal. To summarize, under no circumstances is adipose tissue patterning divided equally over the body (23).

In an earlier study from *Science*, researchers took x-rays of six regions of the body, forearms, deltoid, thoracic, iliac, trochanteric, and lower leg. They then compared this to 12 specific skinfold sites and ranked for accuracy of predictive efficiency for overall fat (13). The findings are below:

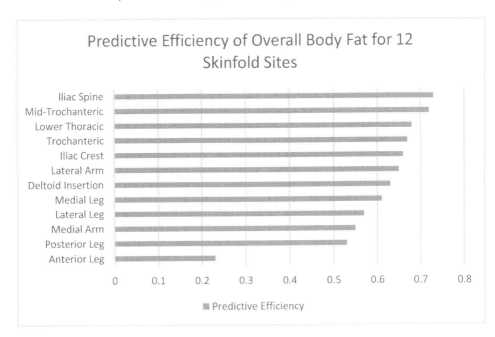

Another early study, this one from the *British Journal of Preventative and Social Medicine*, showed that *"although the best measurements vary somewhat according to the total battery and according to the individuals, the results show that the subscapular and abdominal measurements followed by biceps and either subcostal or suprailiac measurements give the best indication of total fat (17).*

The early study from the *American Journal of Clinical Nutrition* titled **Relative values of different fat folds in a nutritional survey** found the *"The subscapular fat fold systematically evidences higher correlations with body weight than is true for the triceps fat fold (16*

Specific Hormones and Fat Patterning

Insulin

Insulin may be the mother of all hormones. When a person eats a meal, the levels of circulating blood glucose increase as a result. In order to normalize blood sugar, insulin is released from the pancreas. The presence of insulin then signals activation of proteins inside the muscle cells. These proteins stimulate receptors on the liver and muscles to absorb the glucose into the tissues which is then stored as glycogen.

Under normal healthy conditions, the peaks and valleys of insulin release are moderate. Under poor dietary circumstances including ingested sugary drinks, processed carbohydrates or carb only meals, those insulin peaks can be much more extreme.

Here is where monitoring the hormonal effects of food, in particular the Glycemic load, and the timing of those nutrients becomes important. With either an increase in the amount of insulin needed to get the job done or an abrupt saturation of the muscle and liver tissue, the excess glucose has to go somewhere. If you have had poor dietary habits for an extensive period of time, are synthetic exogenous anabolic hormone free, or are not a complete genetic freak, the answer may be between just above your belt line in the form of unsightly love handles or spare tire.

Average blood sugar levels:

Normal fasting before meal: 70-100mg/dl (though some doctors suggest >90mg/dl can be a predictor of pre-diabetic

1 to 2 hours post meal: Under 120mg/dl, with <100mg/dl considered normal 2 hours after eating

Besides the storage of excess glucose and stimulating cells to use carbohydrates as preferential fuel source, insulin has also been shown to effect fat utilization and mobilization in other ways. It has been shown to decrease the activity of the catecholamines and their ability to bind to adrenergic receptors, leading to a decreased ability to mobilize fat cells.

When the amount of insulin normally required to "get the job done" is not adequate, more and more insulin is required to signal the insulin sensitive receptors on the muscles/liver/fat cells to absorb glucose. If enough insulin is not released from the pancreas, the blood sugar levels stay elevated.

> The herb Fenugreek has been shown to have positive effects on insulin sensitivity. In a 2001 double blind placebo controlled study the researchers found significant improvements in blood sugar, insulin sensitivity, serum triglycerides and HDL cholesterol after only 2 months of fenugreek usage in type 2 diabetics (15).

With consistently elevated blood glucose levels, the doors for negative metabolic effects are wide open. Increasing body fat, hypertension, diabetes mellitus, metabolic syndrome, elevated triglycerides, decreased HDL, as well as many other symptomatic diseases can quickly arise with insulin resistance.

Did you know that your Suprailiac (think love handles) and Subscapula skinfold sites may reflect insulin sensitivity and blood sugar regulation?

The 1989 Bogalusa Heart Study from *The American Journal of Clinical Nutrition* found that the suprailliac skinfold was an effective tool in tracking changes in glucose (Freedman 1989). Building on this evidence, a study from the Zaragoza Medical School in Spain looked at the relationship between metabolic complications, in particular insulin dysregulation, and body fat distribution patterning in obese boys. The researchers found **significant correlations between the subscapular and suprailliac sites and insulin/blood glucose regulation** (19).

The researchers also found a correlation between the ratio of subscapular and triceps skinfold measurements and insulin sensitivity. The researchers concluded *"an upper central body fat distribution seems to be first associated with an abnormal glucose-insulin homeostasis (19)."*

A third study on body fat patterning and insulin, this one from 2006, found a significant correlation between fasting insulin levels and the thickness of the triceps and subscapular skinfolds in 324 healthy young adult north Indian males. The researchers pointed out that **the thickness of the subscapular skinfold, in particular, was shown to be a potential predictor of hyperinsulinemia** (29).

The skinfold thickness of the sub scapula has also been shown to be better than BMI and WC in identifying hyperinsulinemia in males and females (20).

In a study from *Diabetes*, a team of researchers measured ten skinfold sites on 7,717 subjects. 360 diabetic and 934 non-diabetic controls were selected. The researchers found that, of the diabetic subjects there was a greater incidence of centripetal fat distribution patterning, which was similar to that of male fat patterning distribution, in both the male and female subjects (10).

The relationship between insulin and other hormones can also have a vast effect on one's physiology. The balance between insulin, cortisol, and testosterone is an oft-overlooked factor. Especially with regards to human health and fat loss. A disruption in the delicate seesaw between these hormones can lead to a cascade of negative effects, ranging from increased inflammation to metabolic syndrome, as the body is no longer able to adequately fight infection and disease.

In simple terms, when one has increased resistance to insulin, there is typically a disruption in the cortisol/testosterone balance. The increased insulin resistance (a stress on the body) elevates the secretion of the stress hormone, cortisol. Or in some cases vice versa, the increased stress levels signal an increase in cortisol, which then signals the body to go into "storage mode" in order to survive the stress. This storage mode leads to an increase in insulin release. The biochemistry is much more complex than this. Now, where does testosterone play a role in all this.

Testosterone is on one side of the pyramidal axis, while cortisol and insulin are on the other points of the triangle.

Cortisol and testosterone have an inverse relationship in which a rise in insulin leads to a decrease in cortisol or vice versa. Well, with the increased stress of insulin resistance, the cortisol levels are constantly elevated, leading to a decrease in the big T.

Estrogen

Estrogen levels are rising in both humans and animals at alarming rates. Did you know that gynecomastia surgeries are rising nearly every year? Did you ever think we would see the day when manziers, mirdles, and mantyhose would actually exist? How about the fact that beer bellies are

> In 2009, the American Cancer Society estimated that nearly 1,910 new cases of invasive breast cancer would be diagnosed *among males.*

beginning to outnumber flat stomachs, hermaphroditic mutated frogs outnumber single sex frogs *(in certain lakes),* and *The View* has higher TV ratings than reruns of the original American Gladiator *(just kidding)*.

One of the major culprits is the hormone estrogen and its family of estrogen mimicking environmental toxins and chemicals. Estrogen is known as the female sex hormone. Formed from the synthesis of androstenedione from cholesterol, estrogen is formed primarily in the ovaries of women by the stimulating actions of luteinizing hormone (LH) and follicle stimulating hormone (FSH). Estrogen is produced in two forms.

First the form known as estradiol, which is formed from testosterone by the enzyme aromatase. The second form known as estrone, is formed from androstenedione.

Androstenedione is one of the precursors to actual testosterone. A male whom does not convert androgens properly to testosterone may have excessive aromatase activity, leading to excessive conversion to estrogen either via the precursor androstenedione or actual testosterone.

Aromatazation of testosterone can lead to unwanted side effects including:
- Body fat accumulation
- Development of gynecomastia (female breast tissue)
- Water retention
- Undeniable urges to comparison shop dishware at Crate and Barrel and Williams Sonoma.

So, what is the problem, besides men walking around with C-cups, listening to Judy Garland, and spending more and more time choosing between periwinkle and purple for their next kitchen paint color. Just a few years ago wasn't this considered metrosexual. Didn't women want their men to be more feminine?

Is Estrogen really that bad? If you are male, a resounding yes, and for females to an extent, well, yes. Phytoestrogens and Xenoestrogens (environmental estrogen mimickers) have been linked to several cancers as well as growth of tumors.

Some of the major problems with estrogen include how and where it is stored, it's accessibility to the cell membranes, and how easily it can actually be produced from its androgen precursors.

Research on estrogen and fat distribution patterns has been quite revealing. A 1999 study out of Japan looked at the effects menopause had on body fat distribution in 764 subjects. The subjects were broken down into 545 premenopausal and 219 postmenopausal women. Upper and lower body bodyfat levels were measured via DEXA scan. The researchers found a significant correlation between body fat partitioning and estrogen hormone concentrations regardless of any increase in overall obesity or aging (18).

A study out of the University of Alabama's Department of Nutrition Sciences looked at body fat partitioning in fifty-two postmenopausal women. The women had their hormones analyzed and body fat levels measured through DEXA scan. The researchers found a decrease in abdominal fat accumulation in the women undergoing hormone replacement therapy. The downside was, with the increased estrogen, they then began to accumulate more fat around about the thighs (14).

A 2012 study from the *Annals of the New York Academy of Sciences* found that women who had gone through menopause had 49% more intra-abdominal fat, 36% more fat about their trunk, and 22% more subcutaneous fat about their abdomen (28).

Finally, 1999 research from Italy looked at the fat distribution patterns of 1075 female subjects. These women were divided into one of 4 groups: premenopausal, peri menopausal, postmenopausal, and sane/rational *(just kidding on the last one)*. The researchers found significantly less leg fat accumulation in the postmenopausal group, compared to the peri menopausal group. This difference was even more significant when comparing the premenopausal and postmenopausal groups. The major hormonal difference between the two groups: Estrogen Levels (12)!

Testosterone

How important is testosterone to your health? Well, a drop in testosterone has been linked to everything from bone health and low back pain to chronic inflammation and cancer. Testosterone plays a role in keeping energy levels up and

Testosterone and fat loss:

- Testosterone has been shown to increase lipolysis by increasing fat cell receptor activity.
- Testosterone blocks the fat storage effects of the lipoprotein lipase enzyme.

inflammation levels down. Beginning in the hypothalamus of the brain, testosterone production is stimulated through a series of hormonal actions. Gonadotropin releasing hormone is secreted from the hypothalamus, which then signals the pituitary gland to secrete Luteinizing hormone. The luteinizing hormone is a signal for the synthesis and release of testosterone.

> **DHT (Dihydrotestosterone):**
>
> - Most androgenic hormone found in the human body, approximately 3-4X stronger than testosterone.
> - The 5-alpha reductase enzyme removes at double bond (C4-5) from testosterone to for DHT.
> - DHT may play a role in balding, acne, and more.

The trouble with testosterone is that its production is not an easy, one or two step process. Testosterone can be converted into DHT (dihydrotestosterone) or aromatize to estrogen. Two other important factors about testosterone are concentration and sensitivity of the testosterone receptors on tissue and how much testosterone is in the form of free testosterone.

So, how does testosterone and lack thereof affect body fat distribution patterns? A 2001 study from *Life Sciences* followed male subjects over a six-month period of controlled anabolic steroid administration. The researchers saw a 53% decrease in testosterone, a 77% drop in Luteinizing hormone and an 87% drop in follicle stimulating hormone. To make matters worse, there was a 45% increase in estradiol (2).

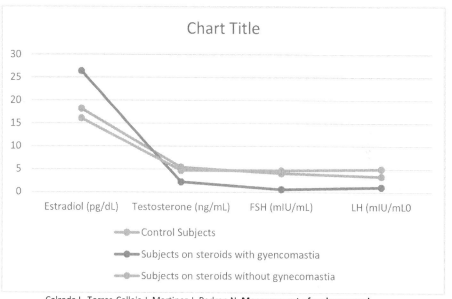

Calzada L, Torres-Calleia J, Martinez J, Pedron N. **Measurement of androgen and estrogen receptors in breast tissue from subjects with anabolic steroid-dependent gynecomastia**. *Life Sciences*. 69(13); Pp 1465-1469. 2001.

The majority of the tissue that became gynecomastia had significant concentration of either androgen or estrogen receptors. The researchers theorized the development of gynecomastia was potentially dependent on three variables:

- ➢ Anabolic steroid administration for prolonged periods may cause an excess of circulating estrogens, perhaps through the conversion of testosterone to estrogen;
- ➢ A predominant estrogen effect on the breast may produce breast enlargement;

> The presence of estradiol and androgen receptors in gynecomastia tissue suggests that gynecomastia is a hormone dependent event

A separate study found that men with low testosterone stored more fat in their lower body during a six-hour period post-meal. Men with healthy testosterone were burn not only burned more fat during that period of time, but they also had a tendency to store less in their lower body fat depots (24).

Growth Hormone

Known as a peptide hormone, growth hormone is capable of increasing muscle mass, decreasing body fat, healing structural tissue, decreasing inflammation, improving cardiovascular function, basically, fending off the physical symptoms of aging. In excess, though, it can lead to cancer, cardiovascular risks, and diabetes.

Secreted from the anterior pituitary gland, growth hormone production is stimulated by Growth Hormone Releasing Hormone (GHRH) produced in the hypothalamus (*somatostatin is the hormone released from the hypothalamus that inhibits growth hormone production*). Once growth hormone has been released, it travels to the liver. There it stimulates the liver to secrete a hormone called Insulin like Growth Factor-1 (*IGF-1 or somatomedin*), which has a similar chemical structure to insulin.

Growth hormone can affect the mobilization of fat cells as GH and IGf-1 receptors are found on the fat cells in your body. When these receptors are activated, they in turn send a signal to begin breakdown of fat so it can be used a fuel.

The body has alpha and beta adrenergic receptors, which are the receptors on the cells responsible for regulation of lipolysis, or fat cell mobilization. They are triggered into action by the catecholamines, epinephrine and norepinephrine. The alpha receptors inhibit fat cell mobilization while the beta receptors stimulate it. Growth hormone stimulates the beta receptors, increasing their responsiveness to the catecholamines.

With regards to fat accumulation, studies have shown that a decrease in growth hormone can lead to an increase in body fat and obesity. In a 1999 study, researchers looked at the effects discontinuing growth hormone therapy had on body composition in 10 growth hormone deficient subjects. During the initial 3 months of stoppage, the subjects had the greatest increases in subcutaneous fat accumulation. Over the 12-month period, the researchers saw a 48% increase in intra-abdominal fat mass (27).

A second study, this one from 1981, in the *American Journal of Clinical Nutrition*, found that the knee and calf skinfold measurements were the most effective skinfold sites for determining growth hormone deficiencies in children with growth problems. They also found the greatest discrepancy in the abdomen skinfold measurement site, with the measurement more than double the thickness in growth hormone deficient subjects (25). The findings are below:

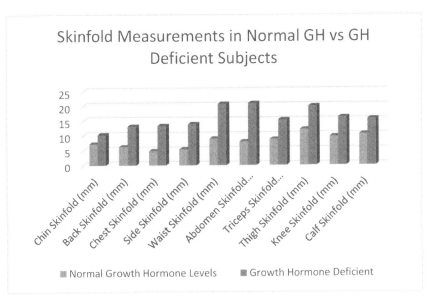

Satinder B, Moffitt S, Goldsmith M, Bain R, Kutner M, Rudman D. **A method for screening growth hormone deficiency using anthropometrics.** *American Journal of Clinical Nutrition*. 34(2); Pp 281-288. 1981.

Peaking in levels around 3 or 4 am, growth hormone is also released in large amounts after a large meal. Growth hormone production is also stimulated by exercise. Studies have shown that higher intensities and lactic acid production are associated with higher growth hormone output (Kraemer et al 1990). Studies have shown that when workouts become stale, growth hormone production levels off.

Cortisol

Cortisol is the stress hormone that stimulates our body to go into protection mode during times of crisis. Picture a caveman whom realizes there will be minimal food in the upcoming winter. His body somehow knows he is going to need to store more and more calories to prevent starvation during the cold months ahead. With this perceived stress, his body goes into protection mode, increasing storage of macronutrients in the cells and body tissue. With this increase of macronutrients, more energy is stored and thus weight gain occurs.

An extremely lean caveman would have had a difficult time surviving the winter months with little fat/energy storage to draw upon when the opportunity to hunt/gather presented itself. So in essence, they became fatter due to the effects of cortisol, in conjunction with other hormones such as insulin. Turn the clock forward thousands of years. The body still works the same, but the availability of food is much different. The problem is that stressors are ever-present, whereas back then it may have been intermittent.

So how does cortisol cause weight gain? After it's secretion from the adrenal gland, cortisol can decrease the action of specialized receptors on cells, called GLUT-4 receptors, which are responsible for shuttling circulating glucose into muscle and fat cells. With the decrease of glucose absorption in the cells, there is more glucose floating around the bloodstream, which can lead to various metabolic conditions.

The excessive levels of cortisol can then create a viscous cycle, in which people can become more stressed as they begin to gain weight, so they eat more crappy food to spike serotonin to make themselves feel better. With more sugar laden foods, comes more insulin resistance, and of course....more weight gain. Particularly around the stomach area, as numerous studies have found excessive "belly" fat storage is strongly correlated to elevated cortisol levels.

A 1994 study from *Obesity Research* entitled **Stress induced cortisol response and fat distribution in women** found a positive correlation between cortisol secretion and abdominal fat distribution (21). A similar study from 1999, this one on men, had similar findings, expressing that cortisol contributed to the subject's greater abdominal fat depots (8).

A research paper from 2003, associated the stresses of a modern society as contributing factors to the epidemic of abdominal obesity (5). One of the reasons for this cortisol/abdominal obesity link is that, as we saw in the previous chapter, visceral fat has a greater concentration of cortisol receptors than does subcutaneous or brown fat.

Excessive cortisol can lead to the breakdown of muscle proteins into their amino acid constituents, to be converted into usable fuel by the liver. With less muscle comes a metabolic slowdown, and with this metabolic slowdown comes stress, and with greater levels of chronic stress comes elevated cortisol levels, and the cycle begins again.

Too much cortisol can be responsible for many physiological and psychological problems including anxiety, insomnia, depression, cancer, cardiovascular risk factors, obesity, Cushing's Syndrome, and many other adverse health effects.

Cortisol is not all bad. As a matter of fact, cortisol is the hormone that helps the immune system to fight off inflammation. Kind of ironic. A hormone, when in excess, can cause inflammation, is actually one of the body's primary defenses against inflammation. Cortisol levels typically peak early in the morning around 7 or 8 am, and drop to a daily low sometime mid-afternoon, roughly around 4pm. It is chronically high cortisol levels we need to worry about.

Thyroid Hormone

According to the textbook, *Endocrinology*, the authors state *"thyroid hormones are extremely important and have diverse actions. They act on virtually every cell in the body to alter gene transcription: under- or over-production of these hormones has potent effects (22)"*.

Thyroid hormone, actually there are two, thyroxine (T4) and triiodothyronine (T3), are produced in a small gland at the base of the throat, called the thyroid gland. These hormones are synthesized from the amino acid tyrosine, also responsible for synthesizing the catecholamines, epinephrine and norepinephrine. Thyroxine (T4) is known as the inactive form of thyroid hormone, while triiodothyronine (T3) is the active form. In large concentrations, these hormones can increase the fat burning effects of the catecholamines, as they can increase the number/sensitivity of the Beta-Adrenergic receptors (30).

From controlling your appetite, to maintenance of body temperature and energy levels, the thyroid gland is a major player in your overall well-being. It can affect your sleep patterns, metabolism and sex drive. Thyroid hormone has such an effect on metabolism that bodybuilders and figure athletes have found their way to injectable T3 to increase their metabolism, and thus, burn more body fat.

In healthy individuals, roughly 80% of the thyroid hormone produced is in the "inactive" form of T4, while the other 20% is T3. To become "active", T4 is stripped of one of its outer ring iodine molecules through a process known as deiodination. Incidentally, the antioxidant/mineral Selenium plays a critical role in this conversion, as the enzyme selenodeiodinase is responsible for stripping the iodine molecule from the outer ring of T4.

Without proper Selenium levels, this process may become irregular, potentially leading to a cascade of negative events, the least of which is a drop in your metabolic rate. A deficiency in iodine may have similar effects as this is also an important component in the synthesis of thyroid hormones.

Speaking of slowing down metabolic rate, the stress hormone cortisol can affect thyroid production in two ways,

1. Cortisol has receptors on the pituitary gland that can shut down the production of TSH, thyroid stimulating hormone, which basically relays the message from the hypothalamus to the thyroid gland, to produce thyroid hormones.

2. Cortisol can affect the conversion of "inactive" T4 to "active" T3. Corticosteroids and dietary induced cortisol elevations can affect the 5-deiodinase enzyme, which is responsible for converting up to one third of the T4 to T3. With the impairment of this enzyme, an iodine molecule from the inner ring may be taken instead. This leads to an inactive form of T3, known as reverseT3.

Estrogen can affect thyroid hormone as it can increase the amount of TBG, Thyroxine Binding Globulin. When a hormone is "bound" to one of these binding globulins, it may become unavailable for uptake into its receptor cells. Certain foods, especially certain vegetables when eaten uncooked, can have negative effects on one's thyroid functioning. These are known as goitrogens.

Soy, stress, and lack of certain minerals such as zinc and magnesium have also been shown to dramatically effect thyroid functioning. It is theorized that stress can signal the brain to turn down production of TRH and TSH, potentially leading to hypothyroidism.

The Catecholamines

The hormones known as the Catecholamines (epinephrine/adrenaline, norepinephrine/noradrenaline, and dopamine) are similar to growth hormone in that these are also formed from amino acids, specifically Tyrosine and its derivatives. Unlike growth hormone, the catecholamines are catabolic in nature. They trigger the breakdown of tissue/cells to be used as fuel.

Synthesis of catecholamines begins with the amino acid tyrosine. Derived from the amino acid phenylalanine, Tyrosine (from the Greek word "tyros" for cheese as it is found in casein protein) is responsible for the synthesis of the catecholamines, as well as other hormones including thyroid and adrenal hormones.

Dopamine is the precursor to norepinephrine, which is the precursor to epinephrine. Tyrosine is responsible for the synthesis of dopamine, so without the amino acid tyrosine, catecholamine production may be interrupted.

Dopamine the plays a key role in several functions of human health including movement, mood, nervous system activation, pain perception, and especially brain function with regards to reward/motivation systems. Parkinson's Disease and the neurological symptoms associated with it are linked to depressed dopamine levels. Addiction is another dopamine related health consequence, as the ingested drugs can increase dopamine levels, putting the user in a euphoric state, but then comes the crash, and the only way to fend off the rebound effects is to raise dopamine levels again by, you guessed it, taking more drugs.

Secreted from the adrenal medulla, epinephrine is part of the endocrine system. The sympathetic nervous system, which is responsible for the fight or flight response, is where the catecholamine norepinephrine exerts its effects, while the endocrine system is the major stomping ground epinephrine.

From increased blood flow to the working muscles, to decreased blood flow to the digestive system, we have all felt the effects of the catecholamines. Increases in heart rate, body temperature, and even that "adrenaline" rush is a response to the effects of the catecholamines.

It is through the alpha and beta adrenoceptors in which the Catecholamines exert their fat loss effects, specifically the beta receptors for fat cell mobilization. The beta adrenoceptors are broken down into beta-1, beta-2, and beta 3, with beta-2 being found in muscle tissue and all three being found in adipose tissue. The alpha receptors on the other hand inhibit lipolysis when bound to by the catecholamines. It is for this reason that many supplement companies have targeted ingredients that can both "turn on" beta adrenergic receptors and "turn off" alpha adrenergic receptors.

When the catecholamines bind to the beta adrenoceptors good things can happen with regard to fat cell mobilization. On the other hand, when the catecholamines bind to the alpha adrenoceptors fat cell mobilization is decreased.

Catecholamines also play a role in thermogenesis. They have a receptor on BAT cells, which when activated, turns on the body's ability to produce heat and stimulate metabolism.

Leptin

Produced in the White Adipose Tissue (WAT), along with another hormone called resistin, leptin plays a critical role in appetite, hunger and satiety. It lets you know when you are full. Leptin is similar to other hormones in that it circulates through the bloodstream and binds to receptor sites,

> How fitting Leptin is derived from the greek word "leptos", which means "thin".

yet it is different in that it is synthesized in the fat cells themselves.

In the brain, leptin influences the actions of Neuropeptide Y (NPY), an appetite regulating neurotransmitter that signals the brain to decrease metabolic rate or increase body fat storage. If levels of this NPY are elevated, overeating and body fat accumulation may result. With low levels of Leptin, NPY levels are allowed to elevate and vice versa.

In obesity, the sensitivity of the leptin receptors can decrease, requiring more leptin to do the job. Eventually the effectiveness of the high concentrations of leptin is not enough and the system begins to break down.

It has been shown that the obesity can lead to leptin resistance, thus creating a viscous cycle for weigh gain and fat accumulation. Think about it this way, leptin is produced in the fat cells. The more obese you become, the more fat cells you have. The more fat cells you have, the more leptin you are capable of producing. The more leptin you can produce; the more leptin resistant your leptin receptors can become. NPY levels are then elevated, and you eat more.

Leptin also plays a role in the regulation of other hormones. The ripple effect of compromised leptin levels can be seen throughout the body. For instance, leptin regulates NPY, which when left unchecked can increase the production of cortisol in the adrenal glands, through its actions on Corticotrophin-releasing hormone (CRH) in the hypothalamus.

Leptin was discovered in 1994, when researchers tried to identify the appetite controlling mechanism in the ob/ob mouse. The ob/ob mouse is known for it's abilty to become excessively obese due to an unregulated appetite.

Neuropeptide Y

This neurotransmitter is linked to many functions in the brain, including cognitive functioning, energy, and appetite regulation and satiety. With regards to fat loss/accumulation, its actions include signaling the body to store more fat and increase ingestion of food/calories. High stress and ingestion of highly processed food can stimulate the release of NPY.

Ghrelin

Ghrelin is a hormone that signals the body when it is hungry, increasing prior to a meal and dropping after.

Resistin

The more obese you are, the more resistin you make. Similar to leptin, resistin is also produced in the White Adipose Tissue. The more obese you are, the more/larger your fat cells, the more resistin you are capable of producing. The name describes this hormone appropriately because resistin causes insulin resistance. "Resist-Insulin".

Glucagon

Glucagon is a digestive hormone, released when food, particularly protein, leaves the stomach and enters the small intestine. It slows the exit of food from the stomach, making you feel full; acts to raise blood sugar, and tells the liver to pump out glucose. It is one of a number of counter-insulin hormones, including cortisol, GH, and epinephrine.

Somatostatin

Also known as Growth Hormone Inhibiting Hormone, somatostatin inhibits the release of growth hormone and thyroid stimulating hormone. It also shuts down the b-cells, the pancreatic cells responsible for insulin secretion.

Chapter IV

The Battle Against the Bulge

Now that we have identified some of the problem areas and why our body chooses to store fat in those areas, let's look at a few key factors and strategies.

Gender Differences

Back in 1992, Dr. John Gray expressed that *men are from Mars and women are from Venus*. There's no question that men and women are different. They respond to different types of communication. Their brains respond to stress differently. They have different hormonal profiles. Is it any surprise then that men and women respond differently to physical exercise and types of training?

Prior to the evolution of readily available Internet expertise, training advice was found in the pages of magazines including *Muscle and Fitness, Men's Health, Women's Health and Oxygen*. In these publications men were recommended to follow the weight training routines of successful bodybuilders, actors and athletes while women were given a variety of "shaping" exercises, yoga poses and endurance training protocols.

In the gym, men would congregate around the weights while the treadmills, ellipticals and group training studios were generally reserved for members of the opposite sex. Women stayed away from the weights for fear of getting "big and bulky" whereas men were locked into the mindset of bigger, faster, stronger.

Did you know that on average, women produce 10 to 40 times less testosterone than men? The average female does not produce enough testosterone to get big and bulky, even if she was training with the heaviest weight possible. Aside from lower levels of testosterone, women also have lower concentrations of androgenic receptors for this hormone.

While men have the advantage in building larger muscles due to higher levels of testosterone, women may be more adept at tolerating lactic acid and producing more growth hormone in response to certain types of training. It has been shown that women can recover faster from and during workouts than men. Possible rationale includes lower or better tolerance of blood lactate as well as less depletion of energy substrates due to their higher estrogen levels.

Women also respond differently to sprint training. Studies have found that women who performed sprint training had greater gains in lean muscle tissue than the male subjects performing the same sprint workouts. It has also been found that women had a greater growth hormone and insulin responses to sprint training, which were key factors in the lean muscle gains seen in women who sprint train.

Another gender difference is that of thermoregulation, or the regulation of body temperature. A 2001 research paper found that women not only sweat less than men, but they also start sweating at higher core body temperatures than men. This is important information with regards to hydration and maintaining electrolyte balance in high-temperature training environments.

The Balance Between Anabolic and Catabolic Hormones

Anabolism, in essence is the building, rebuilding, and constructive part of our metabolism. Catabolism is the opposite, in which breaking down of molecules and tissue occurs. Anabolic hormones include testosterone, growth hormone, IGF-1, and insulin while catabolic hormones include Cortisol, glucagon, and the catecholamines.

Supplements

Controversies aside, it looks like Victor Conti was on to something when he promoted ZMA as a testosterone/anabolic agent performance booster. The combination of both zinc and magnesium can have significant positive effects on both lowering cortisol and raising testosterone in zinc or magnesium deficient individuals.

Magnesium

A 2011 study looked at the effects 10mg/kg for 4-weeks of magnesium supplementation had on testosterone levels in tae kwon do athletes and sedentary subjects. Subjects had their testosterone levels evaluated at rest before and after supplementation and after a workout before and after supplementation. The researchers found increases in free and total testosterone in both sedentary and hard training athletes (11).

A separate study from 2011 looked at the relationship between magnesium and testosterone in older men. The researchers found a positive correlation not only between magnesium levels and testosterone, but they also found a correlation between magnesium and IGF-1 levels (36).

A third study on magnesium looked at the effects magnesium had on sex hormone binding globulin and free testosterone. The researchers found that the higher the magnesium levels, the lower sex hormone binding globulin's affinity for binding free testosterone. In simple terms; the greater the magnesium levels the greater the amount of free, bio-available testosterone (13).

Another positive effect on testosterone levels is magnesium's effects on vitamin D. Magnesium can activate the enzymes that play a role in the body's ability to convert vitamin D to its active form (14).

Now that we have seen magnesium's positive effects on testosterone, let's look at how the mineral impacts the stress hormone cortisol. Magnesium has been shown in research to play a role in cortisol regulation/management (44). It has also been shown to improve quality of sleep, positively impacting the sympathetic nervous system allowing subjects to relax (41).

Forms of magnesium include:

- **Magnesium Arginate:** Form of magnesium that can enhance blood flow efficiency.

- **Magnesium Aspartate:** Has been used in the treatment of **migraines** and has potential heart health benefits.

- **Magnesium Carbonate:** Otherwise known as chalk, used as an antacid, drying agent, laxative, and as a food additive known as E504.

- **Magnesium Chloride:** Effective magnesium for excretion of toxins and production of stomach acid.

- **Magnesium Citrate:** Most absorbable form of magnesium.

- **Magnesium Fumarate:** Form of magnesium that plays a role in **energy production and stress relief**.

- **Magnesium Glycinate:** great magnesium for <u>relaxing muscles</u>.

- **Magnesium Lactate:** Magnesium that is associated with glucose metabolism, and healthy teeth and bones.

- **Magnesium Malate:** Good magnesium to take during the day if daytime fatigue is an issue.

- **Magnesium Orotate:** Magnesium that can **<u>enter into the cells</u>** to promote overall health and wellness.

- **Magnesium Oxide:** common use as a laxative (milk of magnesia).

- **Magnesium Sulfate:** Otherwise known as Epsom salt, commonly used for relaxation and reducing soreness and swelling in muscles.

- **Magnesium Taurate:** **<u>One of the most absorbable form of magnesium</u>**, this form of magnesium can play a role in the regulation of neurotransmitters as well as heart health.

- **Magnesium Threonate:** The only form of magnesium that can cross the blood-brain barrier and increase magnesium levels in the brain, has been linked to improvements in cognitive functioning. It can be found under the patent name Magtein.

Zinc

Similar to magnesium, zinc can also have positive effects on testosterone in zinc deficient individuals. A 1996 study looked at the relationship between testosterone and zinc levels in forty male subjects. The same study also looked at the effects three to six months of zinc gluconate supplementation had on 9 zinc deficient males. The researchers found testosterone levels to nearly double in the 9 zinc deficient males after six months of supplementation, jumping from 8.3nmol/L to 16.0nmol/L. The researchers concluded that there was a significant correlation between zinc levels and testosterone in men (43).

Vitamin D

Vitamin D plays a role in the production of testosterone. One study had men supplement with vitamin D for one year and saw a significant increase in testosterone. A 2011 study had 165 subjects take 3,332 IU vitamin D/day or a placebo for one year. Not only was there a significant increase in vitamin D levels, but both free and total testosterone levels increased in the subjects taking vitamin D (42).

A separate study, this one from 2010, measured vitamin D (25(OH)D), sex hormone binding globulin, and testosterone in nearly 2300 men. The researchers found that men with healthy to normal levels of vitamin D had lower levels of sex hormone binding globulin and higher levels of testosterone. Particularly interesting were the findings with regards to testosterone and the time of year. The researchers found the lowest testosterone levels in March, while the highest levels were in August (58). After winter, in which we spend more time indoors, testosterone levels were lowest. After the summer, in which many people are outside enjoying the sun, testosterone levels were highest.

D Aspartic Acid

A 2012 study saw a 30-60% increase in testosterone when infertile male subjects supplemented with 2.66 grams of the amino acid D-aspartic acid for 90 days (12).

A 2008 study set out to see the effects 12 days of 3.12 g of D-aspartate supplementation had on luteinizing hormone and testosterone. The researchers found an increase in the synthesis and release of luteinizing hormone. They also saw a 42% increase in testosterone levels (51).

Ashwagandha

In a 2013 study, forty-six male subjects received either 675mg Ashwagandha TID or placebo for 90 days. The researchers found a 17% increase in testosterone to go along with a 167% increase in sperm count in the men taking the Ashwagandha (2).

A 2015 double-blind, placebo-controlled study had 57 men break up into either placebo or 600mg/day Ashwagandha group for eight weeks. Muscle strength, body composition, and testosterone levels were among the variables tested. The researchers found a 36% increase in luteinizing hormone, a 15%

increase in testosterone, a significant decrease in body fat, and a greater increase in strength (57).

Vitamin C

A 1996 study found that enzyme upregulation resulting from vitamin C supplementation increased testosterone levels (5). Research from 2012 looked at the effects 1000mg/day of vitamin C, for five straight days per week over a three-month period, had on 120 male manufacturing employees suffering from testicular dysfunction due to lead exposure. The researchers found that vitamin C can protect sperm motility and count, testosterone, and testicular function from the effects of oxidative stress (56).

Carnitine

In a 2003 study, researchers looked at the effects carnitine supplementation had on the hormonal response to strength training. The researchers saw positive benefits on the anabolic hormones while the subjects supplemented with carnitine. In particular, the researchers saw a significant increase in the density of the subject's androgen receptors while taking the carnitine (32). Research from 2006 had similar finding in subjects after three weeks of supplementing with 2g of carnitine per day (33).

In 2013 researchers looked at the free testosterone and carnitine levels in 19 hemodialysis patients vs healthy controls. The researchers found a correlation between carnitine and free testosterone levels, concluding *"the present study gives the first evidence that decreased carnitine levels were independently associated with low free testosterone values in male hemodialysis patients (46)."*

Another way in which carnitine can improve testosterone is through its actions on nitric oxide. A 2009 study from the *International Journal of Vitamin and Nutrition Research* found an increase in nitric oxide levels with subjects taking carnitine. Nitric oxide is a key component in vasodilation and blood flow (6).

Loss of Sleep

Did you know that a loss of sleep can lead to a 15% decrease in testosterone? Did you know that a loss of sleep can also elevate cortisol levels?

A 2011 study from *JAMA* found a 10-15% decrease in testosterone levels in a little as one week of sleeping five hours or less per night (35), while a 2014 study from the *Journal of Clinical Endocrinology and Metabolism* found a 21% increase in cortisol when subjects were sleep deprived (15).

In 2012, researchers looked at the impact five nights of sleep restriction had on cortisol, testosterone, sex hormone binding globulin, insulin, serum triglycerides, and more. The researchers had fourteen male subjects get a good 10 hours of sleep for two nights and measured their hormones and other biomarkers. They then restricted their sleep to four hours per night for five consecutive nights. The researchers found increases in cortisol, insulin, and glucose impairment (45).

A separate study on the negative effects of sleep deprivation also found that four and a half hours of sleep led to a decrease in insulin sensitivity, but the researchers also found higher levels of free fatty acids associated with the lack of sleep (8).

Not only does loss of sleep affect testosterone, cortisol, and insulin, but it also impacts the satiety hormones leptin and ghrelin. The authors stated *"adequate sleep duration and quality are important for the normal functioning of daily metabolic and hormonal processes and appetite regulation. It is clear that chronic sleep deprivation has deleterious effects on carbohydrate metabolism and is associated with an increased risk of diabetes. Altered levels of hormones central to appetite regulation, such as leptin and ghrelin, occur in sleep-deprived individuals and, consistent with this neuroendocrine dysregulation of hunger and appetite, a large number of epidemiological studies have identified short sleep duration as a putative novel risk factor for weight gain and obesity (54)."*

The good news is it seems like we may be able to catch up on sleep, at least a little bit. A 2015 study set out to test if our bodies can actually catch up on sleep. The researchers found that after just three nights of catch up sleep subjects increased their testosterone levels while improving insulin sensitivity (29).

A better night's sleep

Lemon Balm

Studies have shown that supplementing with 300-1200mg of lemon balm before bed can dramatically improve sleep. A 2011 study from the *Medical Journal of Nutrition and Metabolism* gave stressed subjects who struggled with sleep, 600mg lemon balm in the form of the brand name *Cyracos*, for fifteen days. Not only did the researchers see a significant drop in anxiety, but they saw a whopping 42% reduction in insomnia. Seventeen of the twenty subjects saw a full remission of their insomnia symptoms (10).

A 2002 placebo-controlled, double-blind study looked at the acute effect seven days of supplementing with either 300, 600, or 900mg of lemon balm had on mood and cognitive function. The researchers found significant improvements in mood and stress levels in all three dosages, while attention increased with 600mg of lemon balm. Too much lemon balm, in the form of 900mg led to a decrease in subject's level of alertness (26).

Finally, a 2004 double-blind, placebo-controlled study broke up eighteen subjects into three groups, 300mg or 600mg lemon balm and a placebo, followed by seven-day break, then rotated the groups until each subject got 300 or 600mg lemon balm and placebo intervention. The researchers an increase in mathematical processing with only 300mg of lemon balm, while 600mg led to improvements in mood and stress (27).

> There are many forms of magnesium and each one can play a crucial role in our physiology. Often times magnesium supplements may have one or two forms of magnesium, and these are often the cheapest "salt" form. Finding a magnesium supplement with high quality chelates forms including glycinate, fumarate, taurate, and oratate is nearly impossible. The only product I have seen on the market is Ubermag Px Plus by Poliquin supplements. This high quality magnesium has all four of those chelates as well as tryptophan.

Magnesium + Tryptophan

A 2010 study from *Magnesium Research* found a decrease in sympathetic nervous system response, which led to an increased ability to relax, in subjects with poor sleep quality who supplemented with magnesium (41).

Another study, this one a double-blind placebo controlled study from the 2012 *Journal of Research in Medical Sciences* found an increase in melatonin, a decrease in cortisol, and an overall increase in sleep quality, in insomniac subjects who supplemented with magnesium (1).

The amino acid Tryptophan boost levels of 5-HTP, which in turn boosts Serotonin levels, the calming feel good neurotransmitter. An increase in serotonin can lead to decreased anxiety and nervousness while improving mood and ability to relax.

Hormones and Training

Besides enhanced glucose tolerance, weight training has also been shown to have positive effects on androgen hormone responses. In 1988, researchers studied nine elite weight lifters over a two-year period, measuring endocrine and neuromuscular characteristics. Over that time, androgen hormones rose significantly, indicating a positive hormonal response to the training. The researchers concluded that the intensive training over prolonged periods of time could lead to increases in androgen hormone production (16).

It is important to distinguish between resistance training and endurance training. Excessive endurance training has been shown to not only be less effective at increasing insulin sensitivity, but also more detrimental in increasing inflammatory biomarkers. A 2003 study found that with excessive eccentric training, i.e.; marathon running, a state of insulin resistance can be induced for up to 48 hours after the exercise bout. Possible rationale includes the dramatic inflammation resulting from this form of training. On the other side of the coin, a smart approach to exercise, including proper resistance training, can lead to an increase in glucose tolerance while decreasing the expression of the inflammatory biomarkers associated with excessive eccentric endurance training (30).

Regarding the hormonal response to different types of exercise, in 2004 a research team studied and compared the physiological characteristics of weightlifters, cyclists, and controls. 41 subjects were broken down into the three groups, with the researchers testing serum hormone levels, strength, power, muscle mass, and endurance. The researchers found on average 50% higher power values in the weightlifters, while the muscle mass and strength values were not as significant. Of particular interest though were the testosterone levels among the three groups. The weightlifters had significantly higher testosterone levels than the other two groups, while the untrained individuals actually had higher testosterone levels the elite amateur cyclists (24).

In looking at the results, the higher power output and strength values seen in the weightlifters may be due to the positive hormonal response resulting from their training methods. One could argue that athletes with higher testosterone levels gravitate toward the strength sports, but the study did provide insight on the fact that untrained individuals actually had higher T levels than their high volume, endurance training counterparts.

So which is better, relative strength work or hypertrophy specific training? Each has their benefits. Depending on the individual needs of the athlete, both may be necessary, as each elicits a different endocrine response. Research has compared the hormonal responses of 10 sets of 10 hypertrophy training versus 20 sets of 1 relative strength training. The 10 sets of 10 elicited a much greater growth hormone response, while the 20 sets of 1 led to more positive increases in testosterone (19).

Strength training is very important, not only for its effects on body composition, bone mineral density, cardiovascular health, but also for its positive effects on the endocrine system.

Strength Training: *It's like therapy for your hormones*

Did you know that a 2011 study from the *European Journal of Applied Physiology* found a 40% increase in resting testosterone alongside a decrease in cortisol after just 4 weeks of strength training (4)?

In essence, strength training is like therapy for your hormones. To meet the demands or stress during and after exercise, hormones are secreted from specific organs. These hormones can have either a stimulating or calming effect on the nervous system, with the level of response being specific to the demands of the exercise.

One of the primary roles of hormones is to maintain homeostasis. When we eat, our blood sugar spikes, the liver secretes insulin. When we are met with an acute stress, our body secretes cortisol and catecholamines. When we break down muscle tissue, our body secretes testosterone and growth hormone to rebuild it.

During a strength training workout, a trainee activates higher and higher threshold muscle fibers due to the repetitious nature of lifting heavy loads through the same or similar ranges of motion until fatigue. This places stress on the muscle fibers being worked, initiating a cascade of physiological events including a change in the sensitivity and even number of hormone receptors on the cells, increasing the production of certain hormones, increases in the cells ability to absorb nutrients, protein turnover is increased, and repair of damaged tissue begins.

> *Did you know* that increases in androgen hormone receptors can be seen with as little as two strength training workouts?

Factors including the intensity of the workout, the loads lifted relative to one's individual strength, rest periods, exercises used in the workout, body parts trained, workout and training volume/frequency, age, gender, training experience, genetics etc. all play a role in the magnitude of these responses. In other words, the harder you work, albeit safely and with proper recovery, the better the positive hormonal response.

Overdoing it and under-recovering can lead to the opposite effect. Rather than creating an anabolic environment in which muscles and the nervous system can adapt and grow, a catabolic environment is created. Stress hormones will be elevated, leading to a cascade of catabolic events including decreased binding of anabolic hormones to their receptors, continued protein breakdown, and a decrease in overall adaptation and recovery.

Several hormones are effected by the physiological demands and stress of weight training. Let's look at a few:

Testosterone

Testosterone, from the German word, *Testosteron*, is regarded as the most potent naturally occurring androgen hormone, due to Its positive impact on muscle growth and strength.

Testosterone is usually found in either it bound state or it's free state. Less than 5% of one's total testosterone is normally found in the free state, with the rest being bound to binding globulins, including Sex Hormone Binding Globulin, or SHBG.

The free testosterone has the greatest impact on promoting anabolic responses, including protein turnover/synthesis, muscle growth, and recovery.

Testosterone levels are usually highest in the early morning upon waking then tend to drop through the day.

So how exactly does this happen? Testosterone can actually bind to both the receptors inside the cell, known as the nuclear androgen receptor, as well as receptors outside of the cell on the cell membrane. Binding to the nuclear

androgen receptor can lead to protein synthesis, while binding to the receptors on the membrane itself may have an impact on contractile elements of the muscle fiber.

Heavy resistance training at roughly 85-95% 1RM, using large muscle group exercises, with short to moderate rest intervals at moderate to high volume has been shown to have the greatest training related impact on testosterone levels. While endurance training can also lead to a slight increase in

testosterone levels, it comes at a price: high levels of oxidative stress and increases in catabolic hormones. These can actually lead to a decrease in muscle mass and strength.

Resistance training can also have a significant positive impact on androgen receptor content, increasing it for up to 72 hours post workout. Immediately post workout though, strength training may have the opposite effect on receptor content. To avoid this, consuming a protein and carbohydrate meal or supplement immediately after working out may be an effective strategy.

Having chronically elevated levels of testosterone may also have a negative impact, as it may lead to a down regulation in the androgen receptors due to the chronic exposure of the hormone.

Growth Hormone

Growth hormone can have a significant impact on many physiological functions in the human body including:

- Increased amino acid uptake
- Increased protein synthesis
- Increased fat cell mobilization (lipolysis)
- Increased utilization of fatty acids as a fuel source
- Decreased glucose utilization as a fuel source
- Cartilage growth and collagen synthesis
- Immune function
- Growth and much more

Growth hormone is typically secreted in pulsatile fashion throughout the day, with the greatest secretions being during the early hours of the night. Growth hormone secretion can be affected by everything from sleep and changes in sleep pattern, to age, alcohol consumption, breathing patterns, gender, stress, illness, supplements, nutrition, daily lifestyle factors and more.

Different forms of exercise can also have an impact on the secretion of growth hormone. One of the major findings in research is the impact exercise induced lactate and hydrogen ion accumulations have on growth hormone production/secretion. Research has shown that lactate and hydrogen ion accumulation are major stimulators of growth hormone production.

Workouts in which trainees accumulate greater levels of lactate seem to be the key to stimulating greater amounts of growth hormone. Workouts consisting of shorter rest periods combined with moderate (10RM) or higher rep ranges have been found to stimulate the highest growth hormone responses. Super sets, tri-sets, giant sets, compound sets, drop sets, and circuits can be effective strength training methods for increasing lactate levels. Sprint training, sled dragging, and prowler pushing are also effective anaerobic conditioning methods for increasing lactate levels.

Gender can also play a significant role in growth hormone production and response to exercise. Studies have found that men have a better testosterone and androgen receptor response to weight training, while women may be more adept to tolerating lactic acid, and thusly, producing more growth hormone. Other research has shown that not only do women recover better from workout to workout, but they also recover better during workouts, possibly due to less energy substrate depletion due to higher estrogen levels.

Women also respond differently to sprint training. Studies have found that women have a greater growth hormone response, along with a better insulin response, to sprint training than their male counterparts. This may have been one of the reasons the female subjects added more lean muscle mass to their legs than the male subjects. Women also have higher GH levels than men post endurance workouts as well.

Another possible rationale is that women have higher serum growth hormone levels during their menstrual cycle, in particular during the follicular phase.

Cortisol

As testosterone is known for its anabolic effects, cortisol, on the opposite end of the spectrum, is known for its catabolic effects. Cortisol can decrease protein synthesis accelerating the breakdown of proteins into amino acids, which are then converted into sugars for the body to use as energy in times of crisis: Stress.

Cortisol can also:

- Decrease glucose utilization and insulin sensitivity
- Suppress the immune system
- Compete with progesterone at the progesterone receptor leading to estrogen dominance. This can lead to an increase in sex hormone binding globulin which in turn may lead to a decrease in free testosterone.
- Can disrupt the conversion of inactive T4 (thyroid hormone) into the active form T3 (thyroid hormone)
- Can inhibit the production of TSH (Thyroid Stimulating Hormone).
- Can decrease thyroid hormone tissue sensitivity
- Can affect areas of the brain, leading to cognitive health issues and anxiety.

Interestingly, it has been found that the resistance training methods that lead to the greatest growth hormone response also lead to the greatest cortisol response. This in theory could have something to do with the positive elements of cortisol: it is also needed to bring the body back from stress and return to homeostasis.

Not only has long slow distance endurance training been found to lower testosterone levels, but it has also been shown to elevate cortisol levels. Studies have found that higher training volumes equaled higher cortisol levels.

German strength scientist Thomas Kurz recommended using a daily, morning hand dynamometer test as a gauge to determine if athletes were under-recovering/overtraining.

Through its catabolic effects, cortisol also plays a role in overtraining/under-recovering. It has been found that chronic cortisol levels over roughly 800nmol/L may be a sign of under-recovering/overtraining. When we think of overtraining and high cortisol, think of the athlete who engages in excessive endurance training: chronically sick, low muscle mass, low muscle tone, chronic joint pain and injury, low strength levels and little power, and in some cases, accelerated aging.

The Catecholamines

The fight or flight hormones. Epinephrine and Norepinephrine (as well as dopamine).

Released from the adrenal glands, adrenaline:

- Increases heart rate and force leading to an increase in blood pressure
- Constricts blood vessels in the skin, kidneys, and digestive tract
- Dilates airways and increases breathing rate

- Increases the circulation of fatty acids
- Increases body temperature and sweat
- Increases brain wave activity
- Widens the pupils

These actions allow for enhanced blood flow and circulation, leading to enhanced overall nervous system stimulation, and enhanced oxygen, substrate and enzyme transport/activity, leading to enhanced muscle contraction, force production and strength.

As exercise is seen as a "stress" on the body, the release of epinephrine is usually one of the first hormonal responses to occur. Epinephrine release can be a trigger for the release of other hormones including growth hormone and testosterone.

The Hormonal Impact of Different Training Methods

High Rep vs Low Rep Training

As we saw earlier, heavy weight training spikes testosterone levels while keeping cortisol levels at bay, while moderate to higher rep weight training combined with shorter rest periods spikes both growth hormone and cortisol.

Perhaps a case can be made for incorporating both training methods, but in the form of two a day training. Heavy resistance, low rep, longer rest period strength and power training in the morning, and higher rep, shorter rest period, lactate inducing hypertrophy training in the afternoon/evening.

This may give the trainee the best of both worlds: training that spikes testosterone in the am when testosterone levels are naturally the highest, then training that spikes GH in the pm (not to mention the added bonus of another testosterone boost when T levels are starting to drop later in the day.

Large Muscle Group Compound Exercises

Quick question: What muscle group does the deadlift not work? Aside from the Olympic lifts, the deadlift may be the singular exercise that recruits the most muscles, followed by squats. Because of the amount of muscle mass recruitment and overall stress it places on the body, deadlifts performed at low rep (1-5), high intensity (85% +), moderate rest periods, can elevate testosterone levels (59).

A 2008 study from the *Journal of Strength and Conditioning Research* found increased testosterone levels in professional rugby players using lower reps and moderate rest. The exercises chosen may have also played a factor in the increased testosterone. The exercises chosen were squats, bench press, seated rows, and leg press; all compound movements (4).

Two-a-day training

Understanding that resistance training increases glucose tolerance and insulin sensitivity after a workout, just imagine what the effects of two workouts in one day might be. The possibility of an optimal hormonal profile along with an increase in insulin sensitivity twice in one day exists.

National teams have taken the two a day approach with great success by combining several short- duration, high intensity workouts throughout the day. The shorter workouts allow the body to keep cortisol levels at bay while keeping testosterone optimal. Multiple workouts also allow the athletes to train and eat without gaining excessive body fat due to the positive glucose tolerance and increased insulin sensitivity.

In 2007, researchers compared the effects of one a day and twice a-day training in ten nationally ranked competitive weightlifters. After the three-week study period, the two a day training group had twice the gain in EMG muscle activation results, as well as much more favorable increases in testosterone and testosterone/cortisol ratios (20).

On an acute level, the effects of twice a day training can be just as important as the long term effects. Research out of Finland tested those effects. After two high intensity- training sessions in one day, the researchers studied various strength, EMG, and hormonal parameters in the subjects. Though decreases in EMG and isometric strength were seen, increases in testosterone were measured during the second workout of the day, followed by a drop in these hormones post workout. The researchers concluded that acute hormonal and neuromuscular responses could be elicited with two a day high intensity training (17).

The same research team then studied the same eight weightlifters through one week of two a day training sessions, monitoring the same physiological variables. Once again, decreases in EMG and isometric strength were seen, while significant increases in free and total testosterone were seen during the second training session of each day. One of the most interesting findings of this study was the testosterone rebound that occurred. The researchers found the T levels to gradually decrease as the week went on, but after only one day of rest, the

T levels had rebounded back to the baseline levels measured before the training started. If the study had been longer, with T level measurements during the rest and recovery periods, the T levels could have potentially rebounded to even greater levels. It is for this reason that phases of hard training followed by proper recovery can lead to dramatic gains in strength, power, and hypertrophy (18).

We know relative strength training and hypertrophy training elicit different hormonal responses. We have seen that two a-day training can be of benefit for lean muscle accumulation and optimal hormonal profile. We know that glucose tolerance and insulin sensitivity are highly important factors in minimizing body fat accumulation. What else can we do?

Training Efficiency and Olympic Weightlifting

Olympic weightlifting has gained popularity the past few years with the growth of many cross training workout regimens and centers. The Olympic lifts consist of the Snatch and the Clean and Jerk. Related exercises include variations from various start and catch positions. Athletes and strength coaches have used these exercises for decades due to their explosive characteristics and ability to develop triple extension: extension of the hips, knees and ankles. Explosive triple extension may be one of the single greatest movement characteristics separating athletes on the field.

Another great quality of Olympic weightlifting is its ability to actively recruit a large number of motor units/muscle fibers with just one lift. It may be the most compound of compound exercises. When done properly, the muscles of the posterior chain (glutes, hammies, low, mid and upper back, calf musculature) are all activated to initiate the pulling movement. Upon completion of the second pull, the catch involves a deep squat, requiring the muscles about the core, back, shoulders, quadriceps, and hips to eccentrically load the weight and then concentrically drive the weight upward in a front squat.

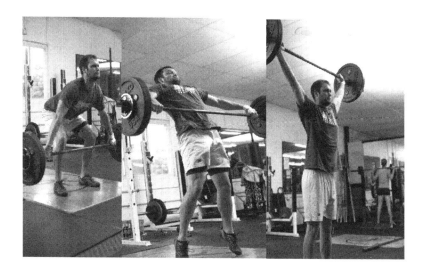

A study from 2007 compared the metabolic effects of exercises with high contraction speeds versus those with low contraction speeds. The researchers had 9 subjects perform squat variations at different contractions speeds with different loads. Blood lactate samples were collected every 15 minutes for one hour after the workout, while expired air was taken before, during, 60, and 90 minutes post workout. The researchers found higher blood lactate levels after the slow contraction training, but the energy expenditure rates were significantly greater during and after the workout with the explosive training group (39).

Not only have Olympic lifts been associated with dramatic increases in strength and power, but their effects on metabolism and androgenic hormone production may be under appreciated. Studies have shown Olympic lifts to have positive effects on androgen hormones and strength gains. From their maximization of motor unit recruitment, to their eccentric-less movement, Olympic lifts are one of the most efficient methods of optimizing strength, power and metabolism.

Another overlooked element of the Olympic lifts is their ability to create and improve flexibility. From the initial starting position, which requires hamstring flexibility and low back mobility, to the catch which requires flexibility about the hips, shoulders, and back, these lifts are an excellent method of actively training transferable flexibility.

Manual Labor

In a three month 2013 study from *Evolution and Human Behavior*, researchers tested the testosterone levels of horticultural tribesman in Bolivia before an hour of intense manual labor, wood chopping. The researchers found that testosterone levels had increased an average of 48.6% after an hour of chopping wood. They concluded *"when engaged in heavy physical activity, testosterone increases, allowing for the rapid muscular performance enhancement* (53)."

Let MRI and Anatomy Be Your Guide

In his groundbreaking 1999 book, *Target Bodybuilding*, world renowned expert/researcher in the field of physiology and strength training, Pier Tesch, released his remarkable research on MRI and muscle activation during dozens of leg and arm exercises.

Training tip: One hour before workout nitrates found in beetroot powder, arugula, turnips, kale, celery, and Chinese cabbage may increase ATP energy production

For years, Tesch used MRI technology to determine exactly what muscles and muscle heads were most active during numerous exercises. This information can be critical in the development of structural balance, strength, and hypertrophy. When combined with a working knowledge of muscle actions, origins, and insertions, trainees can bring their workouts to a whole new level.

Below are a few superset, tri-set, and giant set examples of programming using this information.

Sample Biceps/Triceps Tri-Set

A1: Preacher Curls with EZ Bar (Biceps Brachi: short head of biceps emphasis) X 8-10 @ 4010 tempo. Rest 20-30 seconds

A2: Incline Dumbbell Hammer Curls (Brachialis/long head of biceps emphasis) X 8-10 @ 3020 tempo. Rest 20-30 seconds

A3: Zottman Curls (Medial head of Biceps Brachi during concentric/Brachioradialis and Brachialis emphasis on eccentric) X 8-10 @ 4020 tempo. Rest 60 seconds

A4: Parallel Bar Dip (Medial, Lateral, and Long head of Triceps Brachi emphasis) x 8-10 @ 3112 tempo. Rest 20-30 seconds

A5: Overhead Cable Triceps Extension (Lateral head emphasis) x 8-10 @ 4011 tempo. Rest 20-30 seconds

A6: Straight Bar Triceps Push Down (Lateral and Long head emphasis of Triceps Brachi) x 8-10 @ 3011 tempo.

Rest 90-120 seconds then perform again. 5 sets.

Sample Legs Giant Set

A1: Barbell Back Squat X 10 @ 4020 tempo

A2: Step Forward Lunges X 10 @ 3010 tempo

A3: Box Step Ups X 10/leg @ 1010 tempo

A4: Walking Lunges X 20 @ 2010 tempo

A5: Death March ((walking) alternating leg single leg DB RDL) X 20 @ 1010 tempo

A6: Prone 2 Leg Hamstring Curls X 8 @ 4020 tempo

A7: Leg Press X 20 @ 2010 tempo

A8: Backward Sled Drag X 30 yds

Rest 3-5 minutes

X 3 Rounds

Maximizing Caloric expenditure

When Michael Phelps was prepping for his run into Olympic history, a NASA engineer specializing in thermodynamics questioned how Phelps could sustain such a high daily caloric intake without getting fat/gaining weight, while theoretically burning significantly less calories per day.

> ***Did you know*** that training in the sand can increase caloric expenditure? Research has shown that running in the sand can burn up to 1.8 times more calories than running on a flat surface, while simply walking on sand can burn up to 2.1 times more calories than walking on a flat surface.

The math did not add up. His calories burned through his exercise regimen were nowhere near his calories consumed. He then theorized there must be another factor effecting his caloric expenditure. Then it came to him: water. In particular, training in water well below body temperature.

He found that being in the water and training in the water created a thermodynamic effect, particularly on activation of BAT fat cells, leading to increased caloric expenditure.

Taking this a step further, research has shown that not only can water immersion and training have a compounding effect on caloric expenditure, but cold-water immersion can have an impact on hormones, neurotransmitters, and sympathetic nervous system response.

Cold water immersion

Did you know that the practice of cold water immersion along with focused breathing and meditating may actually alter one's fight or fight response to stress? According to a 2015 study from *Clinical Rheumatology* "*a case study of a Dutch individual Wim Hof, who has developed a training program consisting of meditation, breathing techniques, and exposure to cold to voluntarily influence the physiological stress response, revealed that this individual appeared to strongly activate the sympathetic nervous system and attenuate the immune response in reaction* to controlled experimentally induced inflammation. Recently, a proof of principle randomized controlled trial in 12 healthy male volunteers compared to 12 non-trained volunteers examined the effects of this training program in others, showing remarkably similar effects (55)."

The group that underwent the training reported "fewer flu-like symptoms; showed profoundly increased plasma epinephrine levels at the start of the experiment, followed by a more rapid and profound increase in anti-inflammatory IL-10 levels; and lower subsequent pro-inflammatory TNF-a, IL-6 and IL-8 levels than the non-trained group in response to endotoxin administration (55)."

> **Why are Burpees so challenging?** Total body exercise. Check. How about the effect on blood flow and the heart of standing vertical then quickly dropping to horizontal and vice versa? A study presented at the annual meeting of the *American College of Sports Medicine* showed that performing as little as 10 Burpees as fast a one can have a similar cardio effect to performing an all-out 30 second sprint on a bike. When rapidly moving from supine to standing the body is challenged to keep proper blood flow to the brain. This combined with the blood flow demands of the working muscles of the legs, abdomen, torso, and arms, and there is an even greater need for "rationing" blood to the body and brain.

The Versaclimber

If you have never been on one, this may be quite possibly the most challenging piece of equipment for high intensity interval training *(I am sure many AIrdyne bike enthusiasts would debate this).*

It has been estimated that a high intensity 20-minute interval workout on a Versaclimber can burn up to roughly 22 calories per minute. This estimate is much greater than the estimates of calories burned on in the same time on rowing machines and jumping rope.

> *Interested in making the rowing machine a "little" more challenging,* and perhaps burning a few more calories? Try rowing uphill by elevating the back end of the rower on a small, sturdy, low box. If you really want to challenge yourself, try adding fat grips to the handles as well.

A 1995 research study, this one from the *Journal of Medicine and Science in Sports and Exercise* found the Versaclimber elicited significantly higher max heart rates and oxygen consumption than did the rowing machine or treadmill running [7].

Density Training

Known as EDT, and popularized by strength coach Charles Staley, density training is basically the back and forth super setting of two antagonistic muscle groups for a set duration. The goal is to see how many reps a trainee can achieve in that pre-determined time period.

Target rep range can range from anywhere from 3 to 15 to 20 reps depending on the training goal.

For example, a trainee is working with their 12-15 rep max in the flat semi-pronated grip DB bench press and wide neutral grip lat pulldowns but aiming for 8-10 reps per set, never allowing the reps to drop below 5, for a duration of 10 minutes. The trainee's goal is to achieve as many complete sets of 10 reps as possible, going back and forth between the two exercises with minimal to no rest.

The first workout results may look something like this:

Exercise/Set	Reps Completed
A1: Semi-Pronated Grip Flat DB Bench Press (set 1)	10@ 75lbs
A2: Wide Neutral Grip Lat Pulldowns (set 1)	10 @ 200lbs
A1: Semi-Pronated Grip Flat DB Bench Press (set 2)	10@ 75lbs
A2: Wide Neutral Grip Lat Pulldowns (set 2)	10@ 200lbs
A1: Semi-Pronated Grip Flat DB Bench Press (set 3)	8@ 75lbs
A2: Wide Neutral Grip Lat Pulldowns (set 3)	8@ 200lbs
A1: Semi-Pronated Grip Flat DB Bench Press (set 4)	6@ 75lbs
A2: Wide Neutral Grip Lat Pulldowns (set 4)	6@ 200lbs
A1: Semi-Pronated Grip Flat DB Bench Press (set 5)	7@ 75lbs
A2: Wide Neutral Grip Lat Pulldowns (set 5)	7@ 200lbs
A1: Semi-Pronated Grip Flat DB Bench Press (set 6)	5@ 75lbs
A2: Wide Neutral Grip Lat Pulldowns (set 6)	5@ 200lbs

Ten reps were completed in the first two sets, then the reps began to drop off.

The next time the trainee performs the workout, may look like this:

Exercise/Set	Reps Completed
A1: Semi-Pronated Grip Flat DB Bench Press (set 1)	10@ 75lbs
A2: Wide Neutral Grip Lat Pulldowns (set 1)	10@ 200lbs
A1: Semi-Pronated Grip Flat DB Bench Press (set 2)	10@ 75lbs
A2: Wide Neutral Grip Lat Pulldowns (set 2)	10@ 200lbs
A1: Semi-Pronated Grip Flat DB Bench Press (set 3)	10@ 75lbs
A2: Wide Neutral Grip Lat Pulldowns (set 3)	10@ 200lbs
A1: Semi-Pronated Grip Flat DB Bench Press (set 4)	5@ 75lbs
A2: Wide Neutral Grip Lat Pulldowns (set 4)	5@ 200lbs
A1: Semi-Pronated Grip Flat DB Bench Press (set 5)	7@ 75lbs
A2: Wide Neutral Grip Lat Pulldowns (set 5)	7@ 200lbs
A1: Semi-Pronated Grip Flat DB Bench Press (set 6)	6@ 75lbs
A2: Wide Neutral Grip Lat Pulldowns (set 6)	6@ 200lbs

The trainee has now completed 3 sets of 10. The trainee will aim to keep the same resistance until they have completed all 6 sets of 10 reps in the 10-minute time duration prior to adding more resistance or changing the target rep range.

Concentric Only Training: Prowler Pushing and Prowler Pulling

At high intensities, both of these exercises can lead to high levels of lactate accumulation. Both of these exercises are concentric in nature, lacking the eccentric elements that lead to significant muscle soreness, while taxing the musculoskeletal and cardiovascular systems.

Sample "Legs" Prowler Push/Pull workout:

A1: Prowler Push with arms extended x 30 yds

15-30s rest

A2: Backward Prowler Drag X 30 yds

90-120s rest

X 10 sets

Sample Torso Prowler Push/Pull workout

A1: Standing Prowler Row x 20 yds

15-30s rest

A2: Standing Prowler Press X 30 yds

90-120s rest

X 10 sets

Sample "Arms" Prowler Push/Pull workout

A1: Standing Prowler Biceps Curls x 20 yds

15-30s rest

A2: Standing Prowler Triceps Kickbacks X 30 yds

90-120s rest

X 10 sets

Full Range of Motion Training: Deep Squats

Hartmann H, Wirth K, Klusemann M. **Analysis of the load on the knee joint and vertebral column with changes in depth and weight load.** *Journal of Sports Medicine.* 43; Pp 993-1008. 2013.

Questions answered by the meta analysis:

Why squats to parallel can be bad for the knees: *"Based on biomechanical calculations and measurements of cadaver knee joints, the highest retropatellar compressive forces and greatest compressive stresses are observed at 90 degrees".* In other words, if you stop the lowering phase and transition to the concentric phase at 90-degree knee bend, you are exposing your knees to the greatest compressive stresses (21)"

Why deep squats are good for the knees: *"With increasing flexion, the additional contact between the quadriceps tendon and the intercondylar notch as the tendofemoral support surface (wrapping effect) contribute to an enhanced load distribution and enhanced force transfer. Because lower weights are used in the deep back squat and regular strength training practice leads to functional adaptations of passive tissue, concerns about degenerative changes of the tendofemoral complex are unfounded and unproven (21)."*

Why squats to parallel can be bad for women: *"Women need to be particularly careful during half and parallel squat as* female cadaver knees have been shown to possess 33% lower contact areas of the patellofemoral joint than male samples at 120 and 90-degree knee flexion (21)."

More why parallel squats can be bad for the knees: *"The execution of a half squat cannot be recommended because the turning point is initiated in a knee joint angle amplitude, where the highest patellofemoral compressive forces and greatest compressive stresses occur with only a minor tendofemoral support surface (21)."*

Why parallel squats can be bad for the low back: *"The restriction of the forward knee placement will result in changes to the knee hip coordination with greater forward leaning and ventral flexion of the thoracic and lumbar spine. This evasive movement elicits greater anterior shear forces on intervertebral discs and causes tensile forces on intervertebral ligaments. For that reason, instructions about a restriction of the forward knee displacement have to be strictly avoided. This recommendation is based on a misinterpretation of existing data and should be removed in future practical literature (21)."*

Why you should deep squat with a controlled eccentric tempo: *"The higher the lowering speed in the descent phase, the higher the developing deceleration phase to avoid a dipping movement and hence a rising increase of tibiofemoral shear and compressive forces in the turning point of the squat. For that* *reason, care should be taken to complete a slow and controlled execution comprising a descent phase of 3 to 4 seconds in the deep squat corresponding to an average angular velocity in the knee joint of 46.66 and 35 degrees/sec respectively* (21).*"*

Another reason parallel squats may be bad for women: *"Females possess significant lower compressive strength of vertebral bodies because of their significantly lower end plate cross sectional area than their male counterparts. This means that the female lumbar vertebral is exposed to higher axial compressive stress than a male spine when subjected to equivalent load* (21).*"*

And finally, why deep squats may be better for your ACL: *"In the deep squat loads of 1.16 and 2.27 times body weight accounted for 11.62% and 28.9% of the tensile strength of an ACL in 16 to 35 year olds. The calculated anterior shear forces in the half squat with a load of 1.16 times bodyweight accounts for between 33.29 and 41.56%. Based on these calculations, in deep squats, neither posterior nor anterior shear forces may reach magnitudes that could harm an intact PCL or ACL* (21).*"*

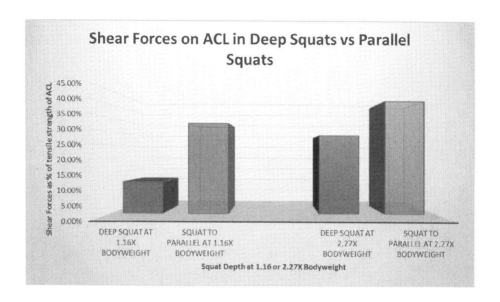

Shear Forces on ACL in Deep Squats vs Parallel Squats

Managing Stress

Tips to reduce your stress levels:

1. **Start the Day off with a Win**
    a. Make your bed first thing in the morning
    b. Drink 16 oz. of water with Celtic sea salt and fresh squeezed lime. This is good for cortisol control and immune function.
    c. Workout. It spikes BDNF production which is good for mood and brain as well as creates a positive hormonal response.
    d. Eat a high quality fat and protein breakfast. These foods have been shown to play a role as modulators of the psychological and physiological stress response.

    e. End your shower with cold water. Cold water has a stimulatory effect on neurotransmitters and blood flow to the brain.

2. **Focus on your ambitions**
    a. Start with a clean space. Clean rooms and work spaces are much less stressful and lead to lower cortisol levels.
    b. Create checklists. Research has shown that creating checklists improves outcomes, decreases mistakes, and improves morale.
    c. Deconstruct your stresses. Dealing with stress is like a game of chess. Realize which stresses require you to make big countermoves.

3. **End the day on a positive note**.
    a. Take Magnesium and zinc before bed. Can help with sleep quality, testosterone, and mood.
    b. 15-minute progressive muscle relaxation. Has been shown in research to significantly lower cortisol levels.
    c. Keep a grateful journal. As little as 15 minutes of positive gratitude journal keeping can improve sleep and decrease worry/anxiety.

*****For more on Stress be sure to check out the book Stress Strategies!*****

Hydration Levels

Did you know that drinking water during 90 minute workouts led to lower cortisol production and a more positive effect on fat burning. It has been found that when muscle cells are hydrated they are more efficient at protecting muscle proteins from breaking down. Fat cells, when hydrated, may also be more efficient at releasing fat.

Alcohol Consumption

From *the Metrowest Daily News /Gatehouse Media* Article **"Alcohol and Fat Loss"** by Jason Shea.

"Unknowingly we may be sabotaging can sabotaging even the best of intentions with some of our lifestyle choices. In a 2008, a study from the American Journal of Clinical Nutrition, researchers tracked the changes in waist circumference of 43,543 subjects over a five-year period. Over that period, the researchers found a 6.7cm increase in waist circumference for women and a 2.5cm increase for men. What was the common variable associated with these increases? (I know I am not going to make too many friends with this one, but here goes): Alcohol intake. The women in this study had an average of 5.5 drinks per week while the men had an average of 11 drinks per week.

In a separate study from the 2003 International Journal of Obesity, researchers set out to determine the relationship between alcohol intake and the effects different types of alcoholic beverages had on waist circumference over a 10-year period. Beer, wine and spirits were the beverages of choice, with nearly

62 percent of the men in the study preferring beer, while roughly 51 percent of the women preferring wine. Perhaps due to the insulogenic effect, the researchers found the group with the highest beer consumption also had the greatest increases in waist circumference over the 10-year period. They concluded, "a high alcohol intake was positively associated with high waist circumference after 10 years in both men and women."

When alcohol consumption was reversed, weight loss became prevalent. In the 2003 American Journal of Clinical Nutrition, 7,735 men aged 40-59 were tracked for a five-year period. The researchers found that those men who switched from moderate to none/occasional drinking showed the highest frequency of weight loss.

So, is it the type of beverage or just the presence of alcohol that leads to weight gain? A 2005 Clinical Review found that of the 67 studies on this topic, 34 showed a positive relationship between weight gain/increased BMI and alcohol, while 21 showed a negative relationship and 12 showed no relationship. This suggests the evidence on alcohol and associated weight gain may be inconclusive. Alcohol's effects on the ability to lose weight and decrease body fat may be another story.

One factor, the majority of studies can agree on is that alcohol inhibits our body's ability to mobilize and burn fat. If you eat a high-fat, low-carb diet, then your body becomes very efficient at utilizing fat as a fuel source. The problem with eating this type of diet while consuming alcohol is that alcohol inhibits lipolysis, or the mobilization of fatty acids for fuel. If you have alcohol in your system, your body's ability to mobilize fat cells to be used as fuel will be compromised. One study from the 1988 Journal of Clinical Investigation found alcohol decreased total four-hour fat oxidation by 79 percent while a separate study found the 24-hour fat oxidation decreased by 36 percent per day.

Because alcohol cannot be stored in the body, its metabolism takes precedent over the metabolism of other energy sources. This can lead to a positive energy balance in which more calories are consumed and stored than calories metabolized and burned. This can lead to fat accumulation and eventually obesity. According to a study from the 1995 American Journal of Clinical Nutrition, even the addition of vigorous exercise was not enough to compensate for poor food and alcohol habits with regards to fat accumulation and lipid balance.

Alcohol does affect individual consumers differently. A 2005 clinical review found that certain factors including the general health of the consumer, the amount and frequency of drinking, diet, bodyweight, genetics, family history of obesity, gender and the presence and effectiveness of alcohol metabolizing enzymes are all important factors in how alcohol affects us individually.

What about the effect alcohol has on your hormones? In a 1988 study, researchers gave 14 healthy med school students alcohol and glucose intravenously. The researchers found an altered utilization of the glucose leading to a decrease in glucose tolerance. They theorized this could eventually lead to impaired insulin response and potentially overt diabetes.

Alcohol has also been identified as a risk factor for abdominal obesity. Potential causes of this include a decrease in fat oxidation, an elevation in a biomarker for increased abdominal fat mass known as gamma-glutamyltransferase, or it could be due to the increase in the stress hormone Cortisol. In research cortisol has been shown to increase with regular alcohol consumption.

Beers are not only insulogenic but one ingredient in particular, the hops, has been shown to have highly estrogenic properties. A serious bender of roughly 120 grams of alcohol or more has been shown to lower testosterone levels by nearly 25 percent for almost an entire day.

From the 1992 Nutrition Reviews, Professor Emeritus from the University of Massachusetts Medical School may have said it best: "Alcohol may not appear as a layer floating at the top of a drink, but metabolically, it is nevertheless more like oil than like sugar."

Nutrition

A simple way of thinking about nutrition when comes to weight loss vs fat loss is: the total calories in vs out determines weight loss while the types of calories consumed plays a significant role in where the weight loss comes from.

With that said, aside from cutting, trans fats, and high fructose corn syrup laden processed foods, quite possibly the easiest way *(for some individuals)* to lose fat is to cut foods that have the greatest impact on insulin: carbs.

Carbs at night vs morning

A 2011 study from *Obesity* looked at the effects of 6 months of carbs at night vs morning in 78 obese members of the Israeli Police Force. The experimental group ate the majority of their carbs at night while the control group had most of their carbs throughout the day. **The carbs at night group had a 20% greater reduction in waist circumference, 22% greater weight loss, and 27% greater drop in body fat %** (50).

A second study, this one from the *British Journal of Nutrition* looked at the effects carbs at night vs the morning had

on our insides, specifically our blood fats and cardiovascular risk factors. The researchers found that the

> **Fat loss tip:** 5-htp to cut carbohydrate cravings 30 minutes before a meal. 5-Hydroxytryptophan is important in the production of serotonin, a neurotransmitter associated with drops in blood sugar and food cravings. Extracted from the seeds of the medicinal plant Griffonia simplicifolia, 5-htp, which readily crosses the blood brain barrier, has been shown in double blind placebo controlled studies to decrease carb cravings and overall food intake, resulting in significant weight loss (9).

carbs in the morning group had higher serum triglycerides and lower HDL than their carbs at night counterparts.

The researchers also found that eating carbs in the morning also sabotaged fat burning throughout the entire day. When the subjects had carbs in their systems, their bodies preferentially burned those carbs as a fuel source. In the absence of carbs in the morning, their bodies burned more fat throughout the day (37).

> ***Did you know*** that as little as 15ml of vinegar per day can improve body composition, waist circumference and decrease serum triglycerides on (31)?

In essence, the above studies are referencing carb back loading, in which carbs are only ingested at the end of the day/evening. This allows for fat burning throughout the morning, day, and early evening, while replenishing glycogen supplies and stabilizing blood sugar throughout the night during sleep. The carbs at night can also increase the production of serotonin to aid in relaxation and winding down prior to sleep.

Intermittent Fasting/Timed Eating?

As of this date (2018), according to personal observation, intermittent fasting seems to work. I have seen lifelong trainees make this one nutritional change, and within months, they have gained significant muscle while losing significant amounts of body fat.

Even professional quarterbacks are now swearing by the benefits of 8 hour feeding periods sandwiched between 16 hours fasts. Not only are they seeing decreases in body fat and

> **Workout Tip:** Green tea extract is a great supplement for a long workout as it can act as an anti-fatigue agent. EGCG may enhance the ability for catecholamines to mobilize fat cells to be used as energy/burned.

increases in muscle mass, but they are also noticing positive benefits with mental clarity and focus as well as a decrease in pain and inflammation throughout their bodies.

The theory behind the lack of pain and inflammation is that when the body is not working to digest and process food, it can put that energy toward repair.

Did you know that the first widely recognized scientific study on restricted diets and their ability to extend life-span was published way back in 1935? In 1935, McCay et al found that rats were able to increase their life spans when they were fed a diet with indigestible cellulose.

The following are a few of the highlights from more current scientific research on intermittent fasting:

- *"the metabolic, neuroendocrine, and molecular control mechanisms governing the biological effects of fasting, refeeding, and caloric restriction are extensive* (52)."

- IF has been linked to lower levels of coronary artery disease and improved levels of insulin sensitivity (22).

- Fasting has an anti-inflammatory effect on the neuroimmune system (34).

- *"periods of fasting can limit inflammation, attenuate pro-inflammatory cytokines and immune cells, improve circulating glucose and lipid levels, and reduce blood pressure* (3)."

- *"Fasting for 7-10 days has shown to reduce pain, stiffness, and dependency on analgesics compared to controls in Rheumatoid Arthritis patients* (40)."

- As a potential alternative treatment for chronic pain, intermittent fasting may play a role in altering some of the neurophysiological mechanisms associated with pain (48).

- *"It may be that alternating periods of anabolism and catabolism, occurring during IF, may plan a mechanistic role in triggering increases in cellular stress resistance and the repair of damaged proteins and cells* (38)."

- Through their impact on brown adipose tissue, *"cold stress may be regarded as analogous to the physiological and psychological stress induced by calorie restriction* (38)."

- With certain nutrient sensing proteins being activated during intermittent fasting/calorie restricting, IF/CR has been shown to improve the integrity of our cellular energy powerhouses, the mitochondria (52).

- Fasting can improve mood. 2013 study had 16 subjects fast while 15 were chosen as the controls. Moods were evaluated at baseline, 6 weeks, and 12 weeks. Along with positive body composition changes, the researchers found significant improvements in mood scores, in particular, confusion, anger, tension, and vigor, in the fasted group only (23).

- *"Clinical observations relate an early effect of fasting on depressive symptoms with an improvement in mood, alertness, and a sense of peacefulness* (40).*"*

One of the major culprits of all of these positive benefits is the ketone body. *"Dietary fasting is known to result in an increased production of ketone bodies, which can be used by the organism as an energy source in the face of limited glucose availability* (38).*"* A ketone is an energy molecule made by the body when there is minimal glucose for energy, i.e.; low carb diet. During low carb

> **Medium Chain Triglycerides (MCTs):** *Think Coconut oil.* MCTs are broken down differently than other fatty acids as they are shuttled straight to the liver, where they metabolized, leading to an increase in ketone body production. Not only does this increase energy, satiety, and body heat, but it may also preserve muscle tissue during intermittent fasting and low carb dieting.

dieting, these ketone bodies are used by the nervous system and brain for energy, while the rest of the body uses free fatty acids as fuel.

The three main ketones are Beta-hydroxybutyrate (BHB), Acetoacetate (AcAc), and Acetone. BHB is not only the main ketone used for energy production, as it is the most abundant followed by AcAc, then Acetone, but it has also been linked to decreased inflammation.

Research out of the Yale School of Medicine found a direct link between BHB and inflammation, in which BHB blocked the inflammasome NLRP3 when administered mouse subjects (60).

In summary, quoting an excellent 2006 study on brain aging and intermittent fasting, *"the main factor that may negate the widespread implementation of CR/IF as an effective geronto-therapeutic is potentially the modern Western lifestyle of near constant work and persistently high stress levels. Hence, to build the society and technological advances that we are used to, we have left behind the feeding patterns of our ancient ancestors in favor of constant mental activity and limited physical exercise. Due to increases in our day to day*

Cinnamon and cardiovascular health: A 2003 study divided diabetics into 6 groups, 1g, 3g, and 6g of cinnamon per day groups and 3 control groups receiving a placebo. Subjects consumed their normal diets. After 40 days the cinnamon groups saw significant positive changes in cholesterol (12-26% drop), LDL cholesterol (7-27% drop), serum triglyceride (23-30% drop) and fasting serum glucose (18-29% drop), with little to no change in any of the placebo groups (28).

activity we have an increased energy (mainly glucose) requirement while our physiology is largely still geared to a feast and famine pattern of energy intake characteristic of our hunger-

gatherer homo sapiens ancestors. This dilemma between our modern society/behavior and our ancient physiology will represent a recurring problem for gerontology for years to come. Hopefully, with our rapidly advancing appreciation of our aging process we will not need to wait for our physiological evolution to catch up with our lifestyle (38)."

Carb back loading + Intermittent Fasting?

Why not try combining both? Eating the majority of your carbs during the last quarter or third of your timed eating period may be one of the quickest dietary modifications to accelerate fat/weight loss.

Chapter V

Putting It All Together

Now that we have seen many of the factors that may play a role in our fat patterning, as well as some preventive strategies, let's delve deeper into an action plan of how to swing the tide in this battle against the bulge.

PHASE 1

First things first: A doctor visit. Getting a full physical with comprehensive blood panel as well as vitamin D and testosterone checked can give valuable insight as to where you are starting.

Taking this a step further, functional Medicine Dr.'s will run very in-depth health screens including food allergy and sensitivity screens, hormonal screen, adrenal health tests, organic acid testing, heavy metal testing, vitamin and mineral deficiency testing, parasite, gut health, digestive tract and toxin screening, and much more.

To find a functional medicine doctor near you, go to the Institute of Functional Medicine's website at www.ifm.org and follow the Find a Practitioner link (*or cut and paste* https://www.ifm.org/find-a-practitioner/).

Now that you have found a baseline the next step is to eliminate the foods that are creating inflammation. Foods that you are allergic or sensitive to will be obvious choices, as are foods containing high fructose corn syrup, trans fats and other processed chemicals. A simple rule of thumb when it comes to nutrition is: if it didn't run/walk, fly, swim, or grow then may be best to eliminate it.

One of the best books on nutrition and food choices is Dr. Jonny Bowden's *The 150 Healthiest Foods on Earth*. He also has a few cookbooks with some great recipes using these foods.

If deficient, adding back the vitamins, minerals, and other nutrients may be effective at this time. For example, if your mineral analysis found that you are deficient in Magnesium, your doctor may recommend a protocol for restoring your tissue magnesium levels. If you are deficient in Vitamin D your doctor may recommend getting more sunlight or set you up on a prescription vitamin D supplement protocol.

The last step in this phase of the action plan is to get a handle on your stress levels and manage the quality of your sleep. In chapter IV we touched on a few sleep aid supplements and stress management strategies. For more on stress check out the book *Stress Strategies* for some great tips on managing stress.

PHASE 2

After we have gotten our baseline health back in order, now it is time to eat and train with the goal of melting fat.

Work. Kids. Sleep. Tired all the time. Oftentimes our workouts are our last priority and can suffer as we are bombarded with the daily challenges of life. Feeling like we have to get to the gym 5 days per week just to maintain or make the most minimal of gains can frustrate even the most die-hard of trainees at times.

In any training schedule or program, quite possibly the most important factor, aside from effort and safety, is adherence. One of the best ways to increase adherence is to have an actual program and track your progress.

The following is a 3 day per week, four-week training program template, designed for the busy parent or employee. Following our discussion on types of training and their impact on hormones, this program contains a heavy day to spike testosterone, a high rep, lactate inducing day to spike Growth Hormone, and a density day in between to address both.

The exercises are written as A1, A2, B1, B2, etc to show supersets, circuits, and exercise order. Reps are written in ranges to allow for nervous system adaptations to determine when you are ready to increase resistance. If you hit the top number of a rep range for all work sets, you have earned the right to increase weight. Tempo is written as 4010 (or 2011, etc) with: **4** (eccentric time) **0** (pause at bottom) **1** (concentric time) **0** (pause at top).

Day 1: Monday: 3-6 rep Heavy Workout

Week	Reps	Exercise Sets	Tempo
A1: Flat Barbell Bench Press			
Wk 1	4-6	4	30X0
Wk 2	4-6	4	30X0
Wk 3	3-5	4	30X0
Wk 4	3-5	2	30X0
A2: Close Neutral Grip Chin Ups			
Wk 1	4-6	4	30X0
Wk 2	4-6	4	30X0
Wk 3	3-5	4	30X0
Wk 4	3-5	2	30X0
B1: Standing Overhead Cable Triceps Extensions			
Wk 1	4-6	3	3010
Wk 2	4-6	3	3010
Wk 3	3-5	3	3010
Wk 4	3-5	2	3010
B2: Seated DB Hammer Curls			
Wk 1	4-6	3	3010
Wk 2	4-6	3	3010
Wk 3	3-5	3	3010
Wk 3	3-5	2	3010
C1: Back Squat			
Wk 1	4-6	3	30X0
Wk 2	4-6	3	30X0
Wk 3	3-5	3	30X0
Wk 4	3-5	2	30X0
C2: Prone Hamstring Curl			
Wk 1	6-8	3	3010
Wk 2	6-8	3	3010
Wk 3	6-8	3	3010
Wk 4	6-8	2	3010

Day 2: Wednesday: Density Workout

Week	Reps	Exercise Sets	Tempo													

A1: Flat Dumbbell Bench Press

Week	Reps	Sets	Tempo
Wk 1	5-10	10mins	2010
Wk 2	5-10	10mins	201
Wk 3	5-10	10mins	2010
Wk 4	5-10	10mins	2010

A2: Inverted Ring Rows

Week	Reps	Sets	Tempo
Wk 1	5-10	10mins	1010
Wk 2	5-10	10mins	101
Wk 3	5-10	10mins	101
Wk 4	5-10	10mins	1010

B1: Standing DB Curls

Week	Reps	Sets	Tempo
Wk 1	5-10	10mins	2010
Wk 2	5-10	10mins	2010
Wk 3	5-10	10mins	2010
Wk 4	5-10	10mins	2010

B2: Overhead Cable Triceps Extensions

Week	Reps	Sets	Tempo
Wk 1	5-10	10mins	2010
Wk 2	5-10	10mins	201
Wk 3	5-10	10mins	2010
Wk 4	5-10	10mins	2010

C1: Leg Press

Week	Reps	Sets	Tempo
Wk 1	15-20	10mins	2010
Wk 2	15-20	10mins	2010
Wk 3	15-20	10mins	2010
Wk 4	15-20	10mins	2010

C2: Step Forward Lunges

Week	Reps	Sets	Tempo
Wk 1	20	10mins	1010
Wk 2	20	10mins	101
Wk 3	20	10mins	1010
Wk 4	20	10mins	1010

Day 3: Friday: 20-Rep Circuit Workout

Week	Reps	Exercise Sets	Tempo					
A1: Deadlift								
Wk 1	20	3	1010					
Wk 2	20	3	1010					
Wk 3	20	3	1010					
Wk 4	20	2	1010					
A2: Flat Fat Grip BB Bench Press w/chains								
Wk 1	20	3	1010					
Wk 2	20	3	1010					
Wk 3	20	3	1010					
Wk 4	20	2	1010					
A3: Chin Up → Supinated Grip Lat Pulldowns								
Wk 1	20	3	1010					
Wk 2	20	3	1010					
Wk 3	20	3	1010					
Wk 4	20	2	1010					
A4: Overhead Cable Tricep Extensions								
Wk 1	20	3	1010					
Wk 2	20	3	1010					
Wk 3	20	3	1010					
Wk 4	20	2	1010					
A5: Standing DB Curls								
Wk 1	20	3	1010					
Wk 2	20	3	1010					
Wk 3	20	3	1010					
Wk 4	20	2	1010					
A6: Barbell Back Squats								
Wk 1	20	3	1010					
Wk 2	20	3	1010					
Wk 3	20	3	1010					
Wk 4	20	2	1010					

More Workouts: If three days is not enough, extra "challenge" workouts for off days may fill the need to workout.

"JUDY"

Try to complete A1-A10 in less than 6 minutes. Then rest 3-5 minutes, and perform a second time. Rest 4-6 minutes and perform a third time.

A1: Power Clean x 5 @ 90-95% of 5RM

A2: 20 yard shuttle sprint X 3 (120 total yards)

A3: Power Clean x 4 @ 90-95% of 5RM

A4: 20 yard shuttle sprint X 3 (120 total yards)

A5: Power Clean x 3 @ 90-95% of 5RM

A6: 20 yard shuttle sprint X 3 (120 total yards)

A7: Power Clean x 2 @ 90-95% of 5RM

A8: 20 yard shuttle sprint X 3 (120 total yards)

A9: Power Clean x 1 @ 90-95% of 5RM

A10: 20 yard shuttle sprint X 3 (120 total yards)

"Century Club"

The objective is to complete 100 reps each of both A1 and A2 (200 total reps) as fast as possible with the same amount of reps per set for each exercise. For example, if you perform 10 reps in the squat on your first set, then need to complete 10 reps of chin-ups on the first set. If perform 8 reps on the squat on the second set, then perform 8 reps of chin ups on the second set.

Times:

Advanced:	< 14:00
Intermediate:	< 20:00
Novice :	< 25:00
Beginner:	< 30:00

Option 1

A1: Barbell Back Squat (bar starts from the floor every set)

A2: Chin Ups

Option 2

A1: Deadlift

A2: Dips

Squat weight suggestions:

Male: 95lbs, 115lbs, 135lbs, or 185lbs

Female: 45lbs, 65lbs, 95lbs, 115lbs, or 135lbs

Deadlift weight suggestions:

Male: 95lbs, 135lbs, 185lbs, 225lbs, 275lbs, or 315lbs

Female: 65lbs, 95lbs, 115lbs, 135lbs, 185lbs, or 225lbs

"10-minute workouts"

The objective is to complete as many rounds as possible of one of these workouts in 10 minutes.

Sample 1

A1: Power Clean X 3-5

A2: Vertical Jump X 5

A3: Clap Pushups X 5

A4: Pullups X 5 @ 2010

X 10 minutes

Sample 2

A1: Deadlift X 10 @ 2010

A2: Split Jumps X 10

A3: Standing Dumbbell Overhead Press X 10 @ 2010

A4: Pushups X 10 @ 2010

X 10 minutes

Sample 3

A1: Squat X 5 @ 2010

A2: Chin Up X 5 @ 2010

A3: Flat Dumbbell Bench Press X 5 @ 2010

A4: Backward Sled Drag X 30 yds

X 10 minutes

"The Millenium"

The objective is to complete 10 rounds of the following circuit in under 60 minutes. 10 exercises, 10 reps each, 10 rounds. 1000 reps.

A1: Deadlift x 10

A2: Flat Dumbbell Bench Press X 10

A3: Chin-ups X 10

A4: Standing Dumbbell Overhead Press X 10

A5: Standing Dumbbell Curls X 10

A6: Standing Dumbbell Overhead Triceps Extensions X 10

A7: Heels Elevated Dumbbell Squats X 10

A8: Pushups X 10

A9: Inverted Ring Rows X 10

A10: Sit Ups X 10

X 10 Rounds < 60s

Nutrition

A basic, simplified way of thinking about nutrition when comes to weight loss vs fat loss is: the total calories in (vs out) determines weight loss while the types of calories determines where the weight loss comes from, ie fat.

Processed foods and chemical additives also plays a role in this. Eating foods from sources that were either killed or grown is a simple rule of thumb to live by when making food choices. Once again, a very simple tip with regards to food choices is: ***if it is not found in Dr. Jonny Bowden's 150 Healthiest Foods on Earth Book, you may not want to eat it.***

Now that we have insight on what to eat, when and how much of each macronutrient should we eat. As we saw in Chapter IV, a combination of intermittent fasting/timed eating and carb back loading may be one of the most efficient methods for dropping weight or decreasing fat.

Quite possibly the easiest to adhere to method of intermittent fasting/timed eating is the 16/8 method. Eat during an 8 hour time period (12:00 pm – 8:00 pm is quite popular) and fast (not including water/coffee/tea) the other 16 hours (8:00 pm to 11:59 am). To back load the carbs during the timed eating periods, carbs can be ingested between 5:00 or 6:00 pm and 8:00 pm.

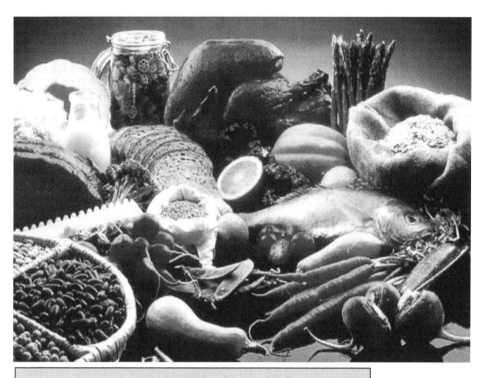

High Quality Fat/Less Carbs Diet

A 2017 study from *BMC Medicine* looked at the effects a higher quality fat, lower processed carb diet had on depression symptoms. The study had 67 subjects, half went on the Mediterranean Diet for 12 weeks, while the other half ate their normal diet for 12 weeks. After 12 weeks, the subjects eating the Mediterranean diet had significantly greater improvements in depression scores, leading the researchers to conclude that *"subjects with moderate to severe depression can improve their mood by eating a healthier diet (3)."*

19 Foods You May Want To Add To Your Diet

Almonds

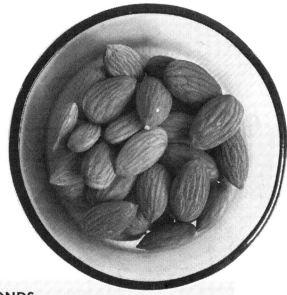

ALMONDS

- High levels of growth hormone promoting amino acid Arginine.
- Magnesium
- Manganese
- Phosphorus
- Iron
- Vitamin E
- Vitamin B2, B3, B9
- 6g protein/oz
- 3g fiber in 1oz
- About 90% of almond fat consists of mono- and polyunsaturated fatty acids
- Antioxidants: resveratrol, catechin, epicatechin, Quercitin
- Lower LDL while raising HDL

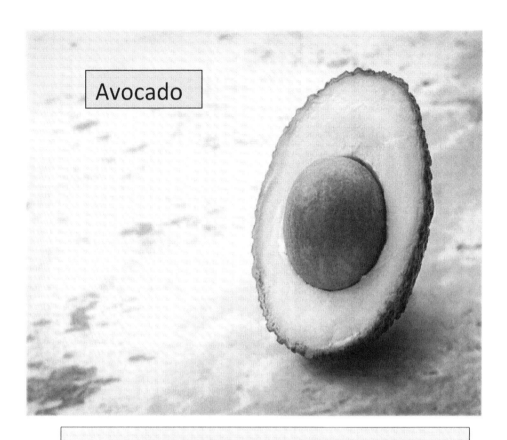

Avocado

- 15g of quality fat, particularly oleic acid
- 4.5g fiber
- Rich in glutathione, a substance that specifically blocks intestinal absorption of certain fats that cause oxidative damage.
- Potassium, copper, and magnesium
- Vitamin C and E
- Vitamin B6 and B9
- Vitamin K1
- Also contain lutein, beta-carotene

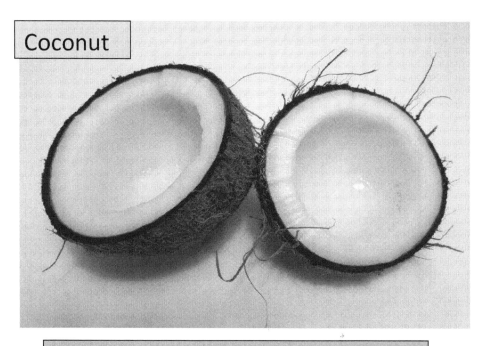

Coconut

COCONUT

- ➢ High in MCT's which in turn increase lipid oxidation
- ➢ Reduces cholesterol, triglycerides, phospholipids, and LDL
- ➢ Improves digestion
- ➢ Contains lauric acid and monolaurin can kill harmful pathogens like bacteria, viruses, fungi, and parasites
- ➢ Breaks down kidney stones
- ➢ Can aid in recovering from food poisoning

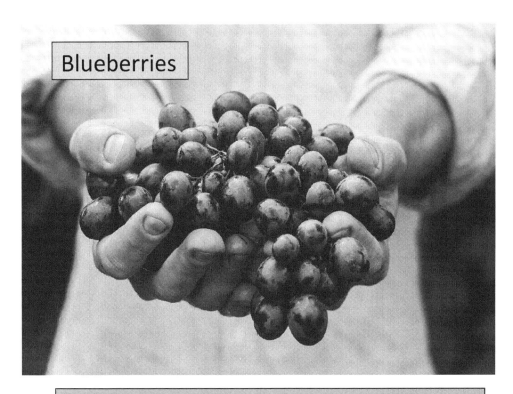

Blueberries

BLUEBERRIES

- ➢ 3.6g fiber per cup
- ➢ High in vitamin C, E, and K1
- ➢ Contains Manganese and Copper
- ➢ Contains flavonols Quercitin and Myricetin
- ➢ Have some of the highest levels of anthocyanin and have been linked to sharper cognition. German researchers tested this by asking 120 people to give a speech, then do hard math problems. Those who had eaten bluberries had lower blood pressure and lower levels of cortisol after the stressful situations.
- ➢ Blueberries have also been shown in studies to improve cognition and protect the brain.

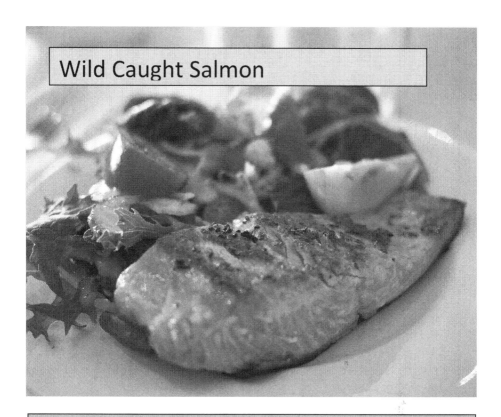

Wild Caught Salmon

FISH

A 2012 study from *BMC Research Notes* compared the cardiovascular response in subjects consuming less than 70g of fish 2X per week to subjects consuming roughly 70g of fish 4X per week. While performing the stressful task of counting backward from 5000 by 13, the subjects consuming the fish 4X per week had lower blood pressure and heart rates during the stressful event (4).

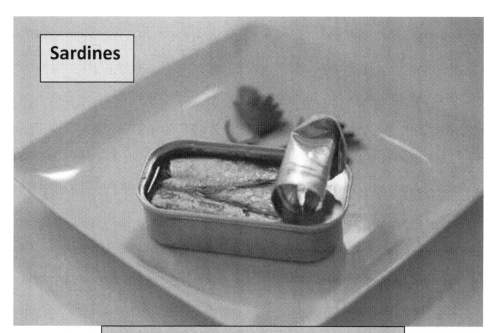

Sardines

> - 36.7g protein
> - 17.1g fat
> - 2205mg omega-3 fatty acids (61%)
> - 101% vitamin D
> - 15% vitamin E
> - 39% Niacin
> - 222% B12
> - 57% calcium (569mg)
> - 73% Phosphorus (730mg)
> - 112% Selenium (78.5mcg)
> - 24% Iron (4.4mg)
> - 15% Magnesium (58.1mg)
> - 17% Potassium (592mg)
> - 31% Sodium (752mg)
> - 13% Zinc (2.0mg)
> - 14% Copper (.3mg)

Broccoli

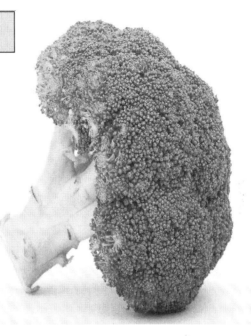

BROCCOLI

- 1 cup 2.3g fiber
- One of the highest vegetables for protein at 3g per cup
- Abundant in Potassium, Manganese, and Iron
- Contains the highest level of vitamin C (165% daily value)
- Vitamin K1 and folate
- Sulforaphane: may have protective effects against certain cancers
- Indole-3-carbinol: also has protective effects
- Quercitin
- Lutein, zeaxanthin and beta-caroten

Cherries

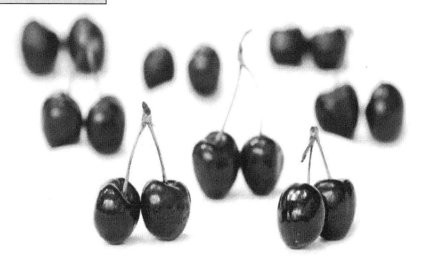

CHERRIES

> ➤ A 2012 study from *Experimental Gerontology* gave 30 subjects extract from cherries broken into two separate servings per day for 5 days. The group consuming the cherry extract had **lower cortisol and higher serotonin levels (1)**.

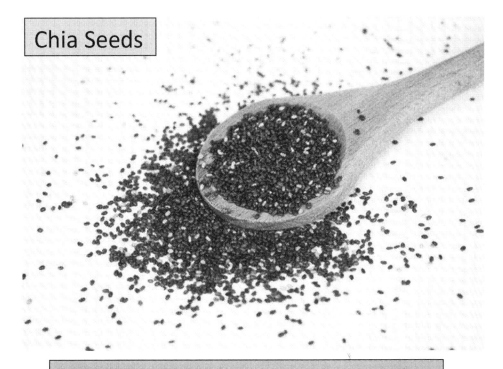

Chia Seeds

CHIA SEED

- ➤ Roughly 75% of the fats are omega-3 fatty acid alpha linolenic acid (ALA)

- ➤ High in calcium, boron, magnesium, phosphorus, manganese, copper, and iron

- ➤ Has more omega 3 fatty acids than salmon

- ➤ 11g of fiber per ounce

- ➤ Contains Quercitin, chlorogenic acid, caffeic acid, and antioxidant Kaempferol

Cinnamon

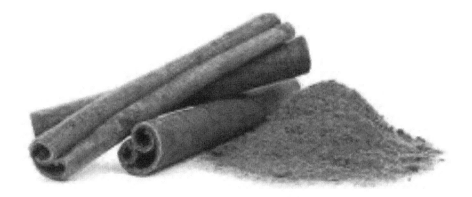

CINNAMON

- High in calcium, iron, fiber, and manganese
- 12 week study out of London found that 2g of cinnamon daily dropped A1C levels in diabetics by 7% as well as blood pressure
- Slows gastric emptying
- Increases insulin sensitivity
- One of the highest antioxidant capacities of any food source

Dark Chocolate

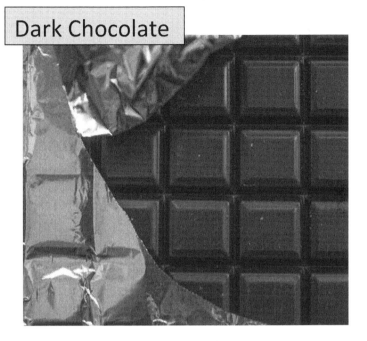

DARK CHOCOLATE

A 2014 study in the *Journal of the American College of Cardiology* looked at the effects 125mg of dark chocolate had on stress levels, salivary cortisol and adrenaline. The researchers found that ingesting dark chocolate two hours before a stressful event buffered stress reactivity and decreased both cortisol and adrenaline levels. In the study the authors also pointed to a *"a 2009 study found that after eating dark chocolate every day for two weeks, people who rated themselves as highly stressed had lower levels of cortisol and catecholamines (7)."*

Garlic

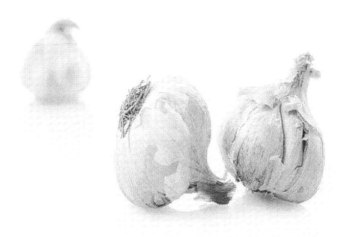

GARLIC

Garlic is loaded with antioxidants and contains Allicin which has been shown to fend off heart disease, cancer, and even common colds. A 2001 study from *The Journal of Nutrition* looked at the hormonal effects of supplementing with garlic while on a high protein diet. The researchers found that garlic may positively impact the anabolic hormonal effect of high protein diets by increasing testosterone and decreasing cortisol (6).

Green Tea

Hintzpeter J, Stapelfeld C, Loerz C, Martin H, Maser E. Green tea and one of its constituents, Epigallocatechine-3-gallate, are potent inhibitors of human 11B-hydroxysteroid dehydrogenase type 1. PLoS One. 9(1): e84468. 2014.

Enzyme 11-beta-HSD-1 converts inactive cortisone into active cortisol in the body. If interrupt 11-beta-HSD-1 in lab animals, they lose abdominal fat

Enzyme 11-beta-HSD-2, converts cortisol back into cortisone.

exposed liver cells to green, black and white tea then injected cortisone to the liver cells and measured cortisol levels. All three teas inhibited cortisol, but green tea had most significant impact.

Compounds epigallocatechin gallate (EGCG) and gallocatechin (GC) were found to be the cortisol inhibitors. "EGCG takes over the spot in the enzyme that is meant for cortisone, interrupting the conversion of cortisone into cortisol."

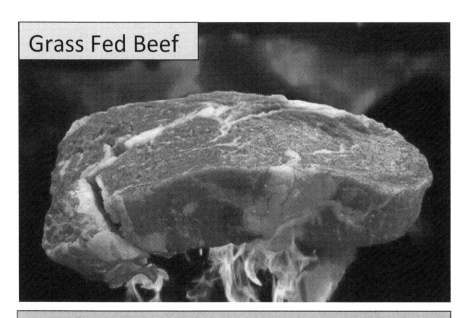

Grass Fed Beef

GRASS FED BEEF

- ➢ Grass fed only have to eat grass 30% of the year. Green fed eat grass, herbs, legumes and other greens 100% of the year.
- ➢ More antioxidants
- ➢ Vitamin C, E, and beta carotene
- ➢ Does not have added hormones, antibiotics, or other drugs
- ➢ Two to four times more healthy Omega 3 fatty acids
- ➢ Zinc, iron, and b vitamins that can help stabilize mood
- ➢ one of the most complete dietary sources of protein with the amino acid profile being almost identical to human muscle

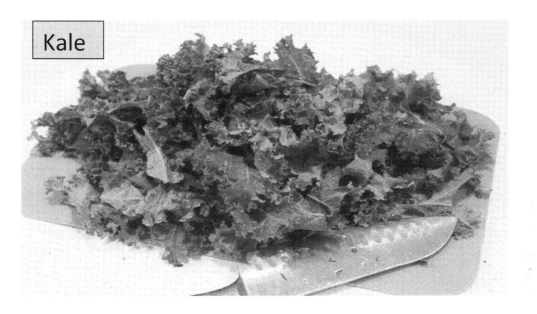

Kale

KALE

- ➢ Contains 206% daily requirement for vitamin A
- ➢ 135% vitamin C
- ➢ 684% vitamin K
- ➢ High in calcium, Magnesium Vitamin B 6, Lutein, and beta Carotene.

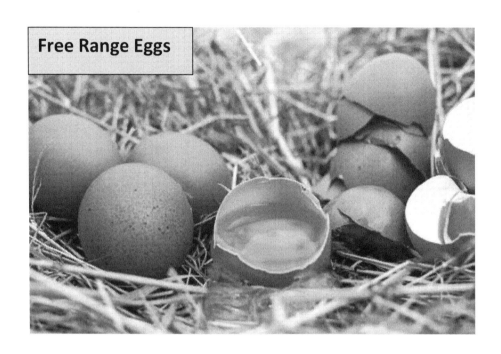

Free Range Eggs

	Vitamin A (IU)	Vitamin E (mg)	Beta Corotene (mcg)	Omega-3s (g)	Cholesterol (mg)
Eggs from Confined Birds	487	0.97	10	0.22	423
Free Range Eggs	**791.86**	**3.73**	**79.03**	**0.66**	277

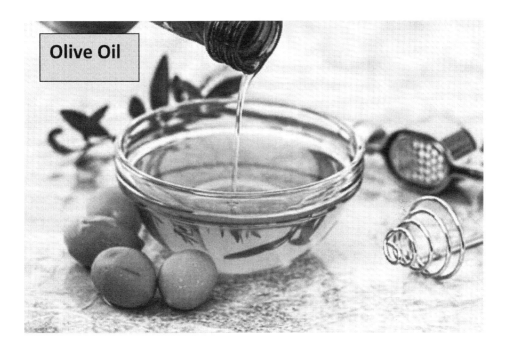

Olive Oil

OLIVE OIL

A 2013 study from the *Journal of Nutritional Biochemistry* looked at the effects a compound of olive oil, oleuropein, had on testosterone and cortisol levels. The researchers found that not only did the oleuropein increase testosterone and decrease cortisol levels, but it also helped the body absorb and retain proteins better, similar to the effects of garlic (5).

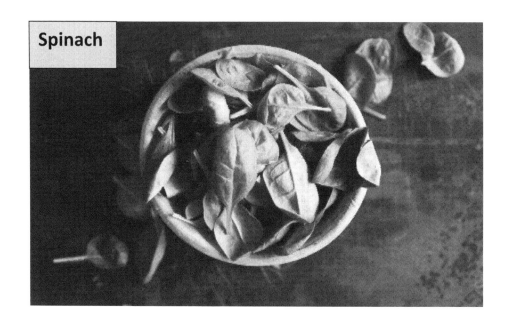

Spinach

Spinach

- ➢ High in vitamin C
- ➢ High in fiber and magnesium
- ➢ Great source of iron
- ➢ Source of folate
- ➢ Source of potassium
- ➢ Source of calcium

Specific Problem Area Workouts: *Glutes*

If your glutes resemble a soggy tea bag or breakfast pancake this section may be for you. Below are 4 challenging workouts that can activate, target, shape, tone, and strengthen your hind quarters.

Workout 1: Unilateral Emphasis Glute/Leg Circuit

Week	Reps	Exercise Sets	Tempo	Rest				
A1: Lateral Band Walks								
Wk 1	12-15	4	2010	20s				
Wk 2	12-15	4	2010	20s				
Wk 3	12-15	4	2010	20s				
Wk 4	12-15	4	2010	20s				
A2: DB Bulgarian Split Squats								
Wk 1	12-15	4	3020	30s				
Wk 2	10-12	4	3020	30s				
Wk 3	9-11	4	3020	30s				
Wk 4	8-10	4	3020	30s				
A3: Single Leg DB Romanian Deadlift Walk (*Death March*)								
Wk 1	20-24	4	2010	20s				
Wk 2	20-24	4	2010	20				
Wk 3	20-24	4	2010	20s				
Wk 4	20-24	4	2010	20s				
A4: DB Walking Lunges								
Wk 1	20-24	4	2010	20				
Wk 2	20-24	4	2010	20s				
Wk 3	20-24	4	2010	20s				
Wk 4	20-24	4	2010	20s				
A5: Unbroken DB or Body Squats								
Wk 1	20	4	2010	180s				
Wk 2	20	4	2010	180s				
Wk 3	20	4	2010	180s				
Wk 4	20	4	2010	180s				

Workout 2: Glutes/Legs Bilateral Emphasis

Week	Reps	Exercise Sets	Tempo	Rest					
A1: 1 ¼ Barbell Back Squats									
Wk 1	10-12	4	3020	60s					
Wk 2	10-12	4	3020	60s					
Wk 3	9-11	4	3020	60s					
Wk 4	8-10	4	3020	60s					
A2: Prone Hamstring Curls									
Wk 1	6-8	4	3021	120s					
Wk 2	6-8	4	3021	120s					
Wk 3	6-8	4	3021	120s					
Wk 4	6-8	4	3021	120s					
B1: Romanian Deadlift									
Wk 1	10-12	4	3030	60s					
Wk 2	10-12	4	3030	60s					
Wk 3	9-11	4	3030	60s					
Wk 4	8-10	4	3030	60s					
B2: Reverse Hyperextensions									
Wk 1	10-12	4	3022	90s					
Wk 2	10-12	4	3022	90s					
Wk 3	9-11	4	3022	90s					
Wk 4	8-10	4	3022	90s					
C1: Weighted Glute Bridge									
Wk 1	10-12	3	3021	30s					
Wk 2	10-12	3	3021	30s					
Wk 3	9-11	3	3021	30s					
Wk 4	8-10	3	3021	30s					
C2: Barbell or Dumbbell Walking Lunges									
Wk 1	20-24	3	2020	90s					
Wk 2	20-24	3	3020	90s					
Wk 3	20-24	3	3020	90s					
Wk 4	20-24	3	3020	90s					

Workout 3: Bodyweight/Light Weight Circuit

Week	Reps	Exercise Sets	Tempo	Rest					
		A1: Body Squats							
Wk 1	20	2	1010	0s					
Wk 2	25	2	1010	0s					
Wk 3	30	3	1010	0s					
Wk 4	30	4	1010	0s					
		A2: Step Forward Lunges							
Wk 1	6/leg	2	1010	0s					
Wk 2	8/leg	2	1010	0s					
Wk 3	10/leg	3	1010	0s					
Wk 4	12/leg	4	1010	0s					
		A3: Arms overhead Walking Lunges							
Wk 1	10-12/leg	2	1010	0s					
Wk 2	10-12/leg	2	1010	0					
Wk 3	10-12/leg	3	1010	0s					
Wk 4	10-12/leg	4	1010	0s					
		A4: Box step ups with knee drive at top							
Wk 1	6/leg	2	1010	0s					
Wk 2	8/leg	2	1010	0s					
Wk 3	10/leg	3	1010	0s					
Wk 4	12/leg	4	1010	0s					
		A5: Walking Lunges							
Wk 1	10-12/leg	2	1010	0s					
Wk 2	10-12/leg	2	1010	0					
Wk 3	10-12/leg	3	1010	0s					
Wk 4	10-12/leg	4	1010	0s					

If your glutes aren't working try this

Glute Activation Sequence Circuit

A1: Static Hip Flexor Stretch x 27-30s (broken down into 3 9-10s static stretch holds, then rest for 3-5s and repeat.

A2: Prone glute isometric contraction X 20-30s

A3: Prone straight single leg hip extension (glute emphasis) x 10-15/leg

A4: Prone bent knee single leg hip extension (glute emphasis) x 10-15/leg

A5: Glute Bridge X 5-6 @ 3035 (5 second isometric contraction at the top)

A6: 3 point kneeling single leg hip extension X 10-15/leg

A7: Lateral Band Walks X 12-15/direction

A8: Pole support squats (hold onto a solid vertical pole/vertical column etc and keep weight through the heels and torso vertical while squatting) X 10-15 @ 3230

A9: Alternating leg step forward lunges x 10/leg

Repeat circuit 2-3 times.

Specific Problem Area Strategies: *Love Handles*

- Look at your Macronutrients.
- Cut carbs, sugars, food chemicals, and processed foods. If it didn't walk, swim, fly, or grow in the soil or on a tree/bush, don't eat it.
- Utilize Intermittent fasting/timed eating combined with carb back loading.
- Utilize the following blood sugar management tips
  - Improve sleep quality
  - Add vinegar to your meals
  - Add Lemon to your meals
  - Add cinnamon to your diet
  - Add MCT oil
- Try the 3 day per week "busy parent/employee" workout from above, keeping the rest periods short.
- Try fasted sprint training or heavy bag workouts.

Problem Area 3: *Belly Fat*

- Try laying off the carb or carb + alcohol laden beverages.
- Manage your nutrition, by cutting carbs, sugars, food chemicals, and processed foods. If it didn't walk, swim, fly, or grow in the soil or on a tree/bush, don't eat it.
- Try Intermittent fasting/timed eating combined with carb back loading.
- Manage your stress.
    - Supplements for cortisol management include reishi mushroom extract, phosphatidylserine, and pantothenic acid.
- Restore your cortisol/testosterone/insulin balance
    - Drink green tea
    - Add quality chelate form Magnesium and Zinc supplements.
    - Add vitamin D supplement that contains vitamin K2.
- Fasted metabolic sprints in the am
- Include Deadlifts, Squats, Chin Ups, Modified Strongman exercises and asymmetrical loaded carrying exercises in your strength training program.
- Make sure you are getting the most out of your ab exercises by including full range of motion trunk flexion exercises, resistance based abdominal exercises, and proper breathing/contacting of abdominal musculature during the exercises.

References

Chapter 1 References

1. Andreasen C et al. **Low physical activity accentuates the effect of the FTO rs9939609 polymorphism on body fat accumulation.** *Diabetes.* 57(1); Pp 95-101. 2008.

2. Bird A. **Perceptions of epigenetics.** *Nature.* 447(7143); Pp 396-398. 2007.

3. Campión J, Milagro F, Martínez J. **Individuality and epigenetics in obesity.** *Obesity Review.* 10(4); Pp 383-392. 2009.

4. Campión J, Milagro F, Martínez J. **Epigenetics and obesity.** *Progress in Molecular Biology Translational Science.* 94; Pp 291-347. 2010.

5. Carnell S, Haworth C, Plomin R, Wardle J. **Genetic influence on appetite in children.** *International Journal of Obesity (London).* 32(10); Pp 1468-1473. 2008.

6. Church C, Moir L, McMurray F, Girard C, Banks G, Teboul L, Wells S, Brüning J, Nolan P, Ashcroft F, Cox R. **Overexpression of Fto leads to increased food intake and results in obesity.** *Nature Genetics.* 42(12); Pp 1086-1092. 2010.

7. Dina C et al. **Variation in FTO contributes to childhood obesity and severe adult obesity.** *Nature Genetics.* 39(6); Pp 724-726. 2007.

8. Frayling T et al. **A common variant in the FTO gene is associated with body mass index and predisposes to childhood and adult obesity.** *Science.* 316(5826); Pp 889-894. 2007.

9. Gerken T et al. **The obesity-associated FTO gene encodes a 2-oxoglutarate-dependent nucleic acid demethylase.** *Science.* 318(5855); Pp 1469-1472. 2007.

10. Hainer V, Stunkard A, Kunesová M, Parízková J, Stich V, Allison D. **Intrapair resemblance in very low calorie diet-induced weight loss in female obese identical twins.** *International Journal of Obesity and Related Metabolic Disorders.* 24(8); Pp 1051-1057. 2000.

11. Hasselbalch A. **Genetics of dietary habits and obesity - a twin study.** *Danish Medical Bulletin.* 57(9); Pp 4182. 2010.

12. Kaprio J, Eriksson J, Lehtovirta M, Koskenvuo M, Tuomilehto J. **Heritability of leptin levels and the shared genetic effects on body mass index and leptin in adult Finnish twins.** *International Journal of Obesity and Related Metabolic Disorders.* 25(1); Pp 132-137. 2001.

13. Labayen I, Ruiz J, Ortega F, Dallongeville J, Jiménez-Pavón D, Castillo M, De Henauw S, González-Gross M, Bueno G, Molnar D, Kafatos A, Díaz L, Meirhaeghe A, Moreno L. **Association between the FTO rs9939609 polymorphism and leptin in European adolescents: a**

possible link with energy balance control. The HELENA study. *International Journal of Obesity (London).* 35(1); Pp 66-71. 2011.

14. Legry V, Cottel D, Ferrières J, Arveiler D, Andrieux N, Bingham A, Wagner A, Ruidavets J, Ducimetière P, Amouyel P, Meirhaeghe A. **Effect of an FTO polymorphism on fat mass, obesity, and type 2 diabetes mellitus in the French MONICA Study.** *Metabolism.* 58(7); Pp 971-975. 2009.

15. Maes H, Neale M, Eaves L. **Genetic and environmental factors in relative body weight and human adiposity.** *Behav Genet.* 27(4); Pp 325–351. 1997.

16. Magnusson P, Rasmussen F. **Familial resemblance of body mass index and familial risk of high and low body mass index. A study of young men in Sweden.** *International Journal of Obesity and Related Metabolic Disorders.* 26(9); Pp 1225–1231. 2002.

17. Malis C, Rasmussen E, Poulsen P, Petersen I, Christensen K, Beck-Nielsen H, Astrup A, Vaag A. **Total and regional fat distribution is strongly influenced by genetic factors in young and elderly twins.** *Obesity Research.* 13(12); Pp 2139-2145. 2005.

18. Martínez J, Cordero P, Campión J, Milagro F. **Interplay of early-life nutritional programming on obesity, inflammation and epigenetic outcomes.** *Proceedings of the Nutrition Society.* 71(2); Pp 276-283. 2012.

19. McCaffery J, Papandonatos G, Bond D, Lyons M, Wing R. **Gene X environment interaction of vigorous exercise and body mass index among male Vietnam-era twins.** *American Journal of Clinical Nutrition.* 89(4); Pp 1011-1018. 2009.

20. Ng S, Lin RC, Laybutt D, Barres R, Owens J, Morris M. **Chronic high-fat diet in fathers programs β-cell dysfunction in female rat offspring.** *Nature.* 467(7318); Pp 963-966. 2010.

21. Rissanen A, Hakala P, Lissner L, Mattlar C, Koskenvuo M, Rönnemaa T. **Acquired preference especially for dietary fat and obesity: a study of weight-discordant monozygotic twin pairs.** *International Journal of Obesity and Related Metabolic Disorders.* 26(7); Pp 973-977. 2002.

22. Ruiz J et al. **Attenuation of the effect of the FTO rs9939609 polymorphism on total and central body fat by physical activity in adolescents: the HELENA study.** *Archives of Pediatrics and Adolescent Medicine.* 164(4); Pp 328-333. 2010.

23. Scuteri A et al. **Genome-wide association scan shows genetic variants in the FTO gene are associated with obesity-related traits.** *PloS Genet.* 3(7); Pp e115. 2007.

24. Sørensen T, Holst C, Stunkard A. **Adoption study of environmental modifications of the genetic influences on obesity.** *International Journal of Obesity and Related Metabolic Disorders.* 22(1); Pp 73-81. 1998.

25. Stunkard A, Foch T, Hrubec Z. **A twin study of human obesity.** *JAMA.* 256(1); Pp 51-54. 1986.

26. Turula M, Kaprio J, Rissanen A, Koskenvuo M. **Body weight in the Finnish Twin Cohort.** *Diabetes Research and Clinical Practice.* 10(1); Pp 33-36. 1990.

27. Whitaker R. **Predicting preschooler obesity at birth: the role of maternal obesity in early pregnancy.** *Pediatrics.* 114(1); Pp 29–36. 2004.

Chapter 2 References

1. Abe T, Kawakami Y, Sugita M, Fukunaga T. **Relationship between training frequency and subcutaneous and visceral fat in women.** *Medicine and Science in Sports and Exercise.* 29(12); Pp 1549-1553. 1997.

2. Alexandrou E, Herzberg G, White M. **High-level medium-chain triglyceride feeding and energy expenditure in normal-weight women.** *Canadian Journal of Physiology and Pharmacology.* 85(5); Pp 507-513. 2007.

3. Ali A, Koutsari C, Mundi M, Stegall M, Heimbach J, Taler S, Nygren J, Thorell A, Bogachus L, Turcotte L, Bernlohr D, Jensen M. **Free fatty acid storage in human visceral and subcutaneous adipose tissue: role of adipocyte proteins.** *Diabetes.* 60(9); Pp 2300-2307. 2011.

4. Astorino T, Martin B, Wong K, Schachtsiek L. **Effect of acute caffeine ingestion on EPOC after intense resistance training.** *Journal of Sports, Medicine, and Physical Fitness.* 51(1); Pp 11-17. 2011.

5. Bjarnason I, MacPherson A, Hollander D. **Intestinal permeability: An overview.** *Gastroenterology.* 108; Pp 1566-1581. 2012.

6. Blaak E. **Gender differences in fat metabolism.** *Current Opinions in Clinical Nutrition and Metabolic Care.* 4(6); Pp 499-502. 2001.

7. Bonen A, Miskovic D, Kiens B. **Fatty Acid Transporters (FABPpm, FAT, FATP) in Human Muscle.** *Canadian Journal of Applied Physiology.* 24(6); Pp 515-523. 1999.

8. Cadore E, Izquierdo M, Alberton C, Pinto R, Conceição M, Cunha G, Radaelli R, Bottaro M, Trindade G, Kruel L. **Strength prior to endurance intra-session exercise sequence optimizes**

neuromuscular and cardiovascular gains in elderly men. *Experimental Gerontology.* 47(2); Pp 164-169. 2012.

9. Cadore E, Izquierdo M, Pinto S, Alberton C, Pinto R, Baroni B, Vaz M, Lanferdini F, Radaelli R, González-Izal M, Bottaro M, Kruel L. **Neuromuscular adaptations to concurrent training in the elderly: effects of intrasession exercise sequence**. *Age.* 35(3); Pp 891-903. 2013.

10. Carswell E, Old L, Kassel R, Green S, Fiore N, Williamson B. **An endotoxin-induced serum factor that causes necrosis of tumors.** *Proc Natl Acad Sci USA.* 72(9); Pp 3666-3670. 1975.

11. Clegg M, Golsorkhi M, Henry C. **Combined medium-chain triglyceride and chilli feeding increases diet-induced thermogenesis in normal-weight humans.** *European Journal of Nutrition.* 52(6); Pp 1579-1585. 2013.

12. Cox C, Stanhope K, Schwarz J, Graham J, Hatcher B, Griffen S, Bremer A, Berglund L, McGahan J, Havel P, Keim N. **Consumption of fructose-sweetened beverages for 10 weeks reduces net fat oxidation and energy expenditure in overweight/obese men and women.** *European Journal of Clinical Nutrition.* 66(2); Pp 201-208. 2012.

13. Dulloo A, Fathi M, Mensi N, Girardier L. **Twenty-four-hour energy expenditure and urinary catecholamines of humans consuming low-to-moderate amounts of medium-chain triglycerides: a dose-response study in a human respiratory chamber.** *European Journal of Clinical Nutrition.* 50(3); Pp 152-158. 1996.

14. Dulloo A, Duret C, Rohrer D, Girardier L, Mensi N, Fathi M, Chantre P, Vandermander J. **Efficacy of a green tea extract rich in catechin polyphenols and caffeine in increasing 24-h energy expenditure and fat oxidation in humans.** *American Journal of Clinical Nutrition.* 70(6); Pp 1040-1045. 1999.

15. Durrant M, Royston J, Wloch R. **Effect of exercise on energy intake and eating patterns in lean and obese humans.** *Journal of Physiology and Behavior.* 29(3); Pp 449-454. 1982.

16. Elbers J, Asscheman H, Seidell J, Gooren L. **Effects of sex steroid hormones on regional fat depots as assessed by magnetic resonance imaging in transsexuals.** *American Journal of Physiology.* 276(2); Pp 317-325. 1999.

17. Farinatti P, Castinheiras Neto A. **The effect of between-set rest intervals on the oxygen uptake during and after resistance exercise sessions performed with large- and small-muscle mass**. *Journal of Strength and Conditioning Research.* 25(11); Pp 3181-3190. 2011.

18. Fenzl N, Bartsch K, Koenigstorfer J. **Labeling exercise fat-burning increases post-exercise food consumption in self-imposed exercisers.** *Appetite.* 81; Pp 1-7. 2014.

19. Foster M, Pagliassotti M. **Metabolic alterations following visceral fat removal and expansion: Beyond anatomic location.** *Adipocyte.* 1(4); Pp 192-199. 2012.

20. Gambacciani M, Ciaponi M, Cappagli B, Benussi C, De Simone L, Genazzani A. **Climacteric modifications in body weight and fat tissue distribution.** *Climacteric.* 2(1); Pp 37-44. 1999.

21. Goss A, Darnell BE, Brown M, Oster R, Gower B. **Longitudinal associations of the endocrine environment on fat partitioning in postmenopausal women.** *Obesity (Silver Spring).* 20(5); Pp 939-944. 2012.

22. Haltom R, Kraemer R, Sloan R, Hebert E, Frank K, Tryniecki J. **Circuit weight training and its effects on excess postexercise oxygen consumption.** *Medicine and Science in Sports and Exercise.* 31(11); Pp 1613-1618. 1999.

23. Holloway G, Luiken J, Glatz J, Spriet L, Bonen A. **Contribution of FAT/CD36 to the regulation of skeletal muscle fatty acid oxidation: an overview.** *Acta Physiol (Oxf).* 194(4); Pp 293-309. 2008.

24. Ijuin H, Douchi T, Oki T, Maruta K, Nagata Y. **The contribution of menopause to changes in body-fat distribution.** *J Obstet Gynaecol Res.* 25(5); Pp 367-372. 1999.

25. Jeukendrup A, McLaughlin J. **Carbohydrate ingestion during exercise: effects on performance, training adaptations and trainability of the gut.** *Nestle Nutr Inst Workshop Ser.* 69; Pp 1-12. 2012.

26. Kelleher A, Hackney K, Fairchild T, Keslacy S, Ploutz-Snyder L. **The metabolic costs of reciprocal supersets vs. traditional resistance exercise in young recreationally active adults.** *Journal of Strength and Conditioning Research.* 24(4); Pp 1043-1051. 2010.

27. Lyons S, Richardson M, Bishop P, Smith J, Heath H, Giesen J. **Excess post-exercise oxygen consumption in untrained men following exercise of equal energy expenditure: comparisons of upper and lower body exercise.** *Diabetes Obes Metab.* 9(6); Pp 889-894. 2007.

28. Mann T, Webster C, Lamberts R, Lambert M. **Effect of exercise intensity on post-exercise oxygen consumption and heart rate recovery.** *European Journal of Applied Physiology.* 114(9); Pp 1809-1820. 2014.

29. Most J, Goossens G, Jocken J, Blaak E. **Short-term supplementation with a specific combination of dietary polyphenols increases energy expenditure and alters substrate metabolism in overweight**

subjects. *International Journal of Obesity (London).* 38(5); Pp 698-706. 2014.

30. Oliveira N, Oliveira J. **Excess Postexercise Oxygen Consumption is Unaffected by the Resistance and Aerobic Exercise Order in an Exercise Session**. *Journal of Strength and Conditioning Research.* 25(10); Pp 2843-2850. 2011.

31. Paoli A, Moro T, Marcolin G, Neri M, Bianco A, Palma A, Grimaldi K. **High-Intensity Interval Resistance Training (HIRT) influences resting energy expenditure and respiratory ratio in non-dieting individuals.** *Journal of Translational Medicine.* 10(237); 2012.

32. Peeke P. **Just what IS an average woman's size anymore?** *Everyday Fitness. WebMD.* January 2010.

33. Pinto S, Cadore E, Alberton C, Zaffari P, Bagatini N, Baroni B, Radaelli R, Lanferdini F, Colado J, Pinto R, Vaz M, Bottaro M, Kruel L. **Effects of intra-session exercise sequence during water-based concurrent training.** *International Journal of Sports Medicine.* 35(1); Pp 41-48. 2014.

34. Rosenbaum M, Prieto V, Hellmer J, Boschmann M, Krueger J, Leibel RL, Ship A. **An exploratory investigation of the morphology and biochemistry of cellulite.** *Plastic and Reconstructive Surgery.* 101; Pp 1934-1939. 1998.

35. Rosenow A et all. **Identification of Novel Human Adipocyte Secreted Proteins by Using SGBS Cells.** *Journal of Proteome Research.* 9(10); Pp 5389-5401. 2010.

36. Rossi A, Vergnanini A. **Cellulite: a review.** *Journal of the European Academy of Dermatology & Venereology.* 14; Pp 251-262. 2000.

37. Santosa S, Jensen M. **Effects of male hypogonadism on regional adipose tissue fatty acid storage and lipogenic proteins.** *PLoS One.* 7(2); e31473. 2012.

38. Schiffer B, Daxenberger A, Meyer K, Meyer H. **The fate of trenbolone acetate and melengesterol acetate after application as growth promoters in cattle: environmental studies.** *Environ Health Perspect.* 109; Pp 1145–1151. 2001.

39. Sedlock D, Fissinger J, Melby C. **Effect of exercise intensity and duration on postexercise energy expenditure.** *Medicine and Science in Sports and Exercise.* 21(6); Pp 662-666. 1989.

40. Soga S, Ota N, Shimotoyodome A. **Stimulation of postprandial fat utilization in healthy humans by daily consumption of chlorogenic acids.** *Biosci Biotechnol Biochem.* 77(8); Pp 1633-1636. 2013.

41. Stephany R. **Hormones in meat: different approaches in the EU and in the USA.** *APMIS Suppl.* 103; Pp 357-63. 2001.

42. Thornton M, Potteiger J. **Effects of resistance exercise bouts of different intensities but equal work on EPOC.** *Medicine and Science in Sports and Exercise.* 34(4); Pp 715-722. 2002.

43. Toth M, Tchernof A, Sites C, Poehlman E. **Menopause-related changes in body fat distribution.** *Ann N Y Acad Sci.* 904; Pp 502-506. 2000.

44. Yardley J, Kenny G, Perkins B, Riddell M, Malcolm J, Boulay P, Khandwala F, Sigal R. **Effects of performing resistance exercise before versus after aerobic exercise on glycemia in type 1 diabetes.** *Diabetes Care.* 35(4); Pp 669-675. 2012.

45. Yoshioka M, St-Pierre S, Suzuki M, Tremblay A. **Effects of red pepper added to high-fat and high-carbohydrate meals on energy metabolism and substrate utilization in Japanese women.** *British Journal of Nutrition.* 80; Pp 503–510. 1998.

Chapter 3 References

1. Albrink M, Meigs W. **Interrelationship between skinfold thickness, serum lipids and blood sugar in normal men.** *The American Journal of Clinical Nutrition.* 15(5); Pp 255-261. 1964.

2. Calzada L, Torres-Calleia J, Martinez J, Pedron N. **Measurement of androgen and estrogen receptors in breast tissue from subjects with anabolic steroid-dependent gynecomastia.** *Life Sciences.* 69(13); Pp 1465-1469. 2001.

3. Clarys J, Provyn S, Marfell-Jones M. **Cadaver studies and their impact on the understanding of human adiposity.** *Ergonomics.* 48(11-14); Pp 1445-1461. 2005.

4. Davidson L, Wang J, ThorntonJ, Kaleem Z, Silva-Palacios F, Pierson R, Heymsfield S, Gallagher D. **Predicting fat percent by skinfolds in Racial Groups: Durnin and Womersley Revisited.** *Medicine and Science in Sports and Exercise.* 43(3); Pp 542-549. 2011.

5. Drapeau V, Therrien F, Richard D, Tremblay A. **Is visceral obesity a physiological adaptation to stress?** *Panminerva Medica.* 45(3); Pp 189-195. 2003.

6. Ebbeling C, Leidig M, Feldman H, Lovesky M, Ludwig D. **Effects of a low-glycemic load vs low-fat diet in obese young adults: a randomized trial.** *JAMA.* 297(19); Pp 2092-2102. 2007.

7. Eisner R. **Skinfold thickness in primitive peoples native to cold climates.** *Annals of New York Academy of Sciences.* 110; Pp 503-514. 1963.

8. Epel E, Moyer A, Martin C, Macary S, Cummings N, Rodin J, Rebuffe-Scrive M. **Stress-induced cortisol, mood, and fat distribution in men**. *Obesity Research.* 7(1); Pp 9-15. 1999.

9. Eston L. **Changes in performance, skinfold thickness, and fat patterning after three years of intense athletic conditioning in high level runners**. *British Journal of Sports Medicine.* 39; Pp 851-856. 2005.

10. Feldman R, Sender J, Siegelaub A. **Difference in diabetic and nondiabetic fat distribution patterns by skinfold measurement**. *Diabetes.* 18(7); Pp 487-486. 1969.

11. Freedman D, Srinivasan S, Harsha D, Webber L, Berenson G. **Relation of body fat patterning to lipid and lipoprotein concentrations in children and adolescents: the Bogalusa Heart Study.** *American Journal of Clinical Nutrition.* 50; Pp 930-939. 1989.

12. Gambacciani M, Ciaponi M, Cappagli B, Benussi C, De Simone L, Genazzani A. **Climacteric modifications in body weight and fat tissue distribution.** *Climacteric.* 2(1); Pp 37-44. 1999.

13. Garn S. **Selection of body sites for fat measurement.** *Science.* 125; Pp 550-551. 1956.

14. Goss A, Darnell BE, Brown M, Oster R, Gower B. **Longitudinal associations of the endocrine environment on fat partitioning in postmenopausal women.** *Obesity (Silver Spring).* 20(5); Pp 939-944. 2012.

15. Gupta A, Gupta R, Lal B. **Effect of Trigonella foenum-graecum (fenugreek) seeds on glycaemic control and insulin resistance in type 2 diabetes mellitus: a double blind placebo controlled study.** *Journal of the Association of Physicians India.*49; Pp 1057-1061. 2001.

16. Gurn S, Rosen N, McCann M. **Relative values of different fat folds in a nutritional survey**. *The American Journal of Clinical Nutrition.* 24; Pp 1380-1381. 1971.

17. Hammond W. **Measurement and interpretation of subcutaneous fat, with norms for children and young adult males.** *British J prev. soc. Med.* 9; Pp 201-211. 1955.

18. Ijuin H, Douchi T, Oki T, Maruta K, Nagata Y. **The contribution of menopause to changes in body-fat distribution.** *J Obstet Gynaecol Res.* 25(5); Pp 367-372. 1999.

19. Legido A, Sarria A, Bueno M, Garagorri J, Fleta J, Ramos F, Abos M, Perez-Gonzalez J. **Relationship of body fat distribution to metabolic complications in obese prepubertal boys: gender related differences.** *Acta-Pediatrica Scandanavia.* 78(3); Pp 440-446. 1989.

20. Misra A, Madhavan M, Vikram N, Pandey R, Dhingra V, Luthra K. **Simple anthropometric measures identify fasting hyperinsulinemia**

and clustering of cardiovascular risk factors in Asian Indian adolescents. *Metabolism*. 55(12); Pp 1569-1573. 2006.

21. Moyer A, Rodin J, Grilo C, Cummings N, Larson L, Rebuffé-Scrive M. **Stress-induced cortisol response and fat distribution in women**. *Obesity Research*. 2(3); Pp 255-262. 1994.

22. Nussey S, Whitehead S. *Endocrinology: an integrated approach.* Informa Healthcare. 2001.

23. Provyn S, Scafoglieri A, Tresignie J, Lume C, Clarys J, Bautmans I. **Critical appraisal of selected body composition data acquisition techniques in public health**. *Public Health: Social and Behavioral Health*. May 2012.

24. Santosa S, Jensen M. **Effects of male hypogonadism on regional adipose tissue fatty acid storage and lipogenic proteins**. *PLoS One*. 7(2); e31473. 2012.

25. Satinder B, Moffitt S, Goldsmith M, Bain R, Kutner M, Rudman D. **A method for screening growth hormone deficiency using anthropometrics**. *American Journal of Clinical Nutrition*. 34(2); Pp 281-288. 1981.

26. Seltzer C, Mayer J. **Greater reliability of the triceps skin fold over the subscapular skin fold as an index of obesity**. *The American Journal of Clinical Nutrition*. 20(9); Pp 950-953.1967.

27. Stouthart P, de Ridder C, Rekers-Mobarg L, van der Waal H. **Changes in body composition during 12 months after discontinuation of growth hormone therapy in young adults with growth hormone deficiency from childhood**. *Journal of Pediatric Endocrinology and Metabolism*. 12(1); Pp 335-338. 1999.

28. Toth M, Tchernof A, Sites C, Poehlman E. **Menopause-related changes in body fat distribution**. *Ann N Y Acad Sci*. 904; Pp 502-506. 2000.

29. Vikram N, Misra A, Pandey R, Dwiyedi M, Luthra K, Dhingra V, Talwar K. **Association between subclinical inflammation and fasting insulin in urban young adult north Indian males**. *The Indian Journal of Medical Research*. 124(6); Pp 677-682. 2006.

30. Wahrenberg H, Engfeldt P, Arner P, Wennlund A, Ostman J. **Adrenergic regulation of lipolysis in human adipocytes: findings in hyper- and hypothyroidism**. *Journal of Clinical Endocrinology and Metabolism*. 63(3); Pp 631-638. 1986.

Chapter 4 References

1. Abbasi B, Kimiagar M, Sadeghniiat K, Shirazi M, Hedayati M, Rashidikhani B. **The effect of magnesium supplementation on primary insomnia in elderly: A double-blind placebo controlled clinical trial**. *Journal of Research in Medical Sciences*. 17(12); Pp 1161-1169. 2012.
2. Ambive V, Langade D, Dongre S, Aptikar P, Kulkarni M, Dongre A. **Clinical evaluation of the spermatogenic activity of the root extract of Ashwagandha (Withania Somnifera) in Oligospermic Males: A Pilot Study.** *Evidence Based Complementary and Alternative Medicine*. 2013.
3. Aly S. **Role of intermittent fasting on improving health and reducing diseases**. *International Journal of Health Sciences*. 8(3); Editorial. 2014.
4. Beaven C, Gill N, Cook C. **Salivary testosterone and cortisol responses in professional rugby players after four resistance exercise protocols**. *Journal of Strength and Conditioning Research*. 22(2); Pp 426-432. 2008.
5. Biswas N, Chaudhuri A, Sarker M, Biswas R. **Effect of ascorbic acid on in vitro synthesis of testosterone in rat testis**. *Indian Journal of Experimental Biology*. 34(6); Pp 612-613. 1996.
6. Bloomer R, Tschume L, Smith W. **Glycine propionyl-L-carnitine modulates lipid peroxidation and nitric oxide in human subjects**. *International Journal of Vitamin and Nutrition Research*. 79(3); Pp 131-141. 2009.
7. Brahler C, Blank S. **Versaclimbing elicits higher VO2max than does treadmill running or rowing ergometry**. *Medicine and Science in Sports and Exercise*. 27(2); Pp 249-254. 1995.
8. Broussard J, Chapotot F, Abraham V, Day A, Delebecque F, Whitmore H, Tasali E. **Sleep restriction increases free fatty acids in healthy men**. *Diabetologia*. 48(4); Pp 791-798. 2015.
9. Cangiano C, Labiano A, Del Ben M, Preziosa I, Angelico F, Cascino A, Rossi-Fanelli F. **Effects of oral 5-hydroxy-tryptophan on energy intake and macronutrient selection in non-insulin dependent diabetic patients**. *International Journal of Obesity and Related Metabolic Disorders*. 22(7); Pp 648-654. 1998.
10. Cases J, Ibarro A, Feuillere N, Roller M, Sukkar S. **Pilot trial of Melissa officinalis L. leaf extract in the treatment of volunteers suffering from mild to moderate anxiety disorders and sleep disturbances**. *Medical Journal of Nutrition and Metabolism*. 4(3); Pp 211-218. 2011.
11. Cinar V, Polat Y, Baltaci A, Mobulkoc R. **Effects of magnesium supplementation on testosterone levels of athletes and sedentary**

subjects at rest and after exhaustion. *Biol Trac Elem Res.* 140(1); Pp 18-23. 2010.

12. D'Aniello G, Ronsini S, Notari T, Grieco N, Infante V, Angel N, et al. **D-Aspartate, a key Element for the Improvement of sperm quality**. *Scientific Research (Open Access).* 2(4); Pp 45-53. 2012.

13. Excoffon L, Guillaume Y, Woronoff -Lemsi M, Andre C. **Magneisum effect on testosterone-SHBG association studied by a novel molecular chromatography approach**. *Journal of Pharmaceutical and Biomedical Analysis.* 49(2);Pp 175-180. 2009.

14. Farhanghi M, Mahboob S, Ostadrahimi A. **Obesity induced magnesium deficiency can be treated by vitamin D supplementation**. *The Journal of the Pakistan Medical Association.* 59(4); Pp 258-261. 2009.

15. Guyon A, Balbo M, Morselli L, Tasali E, Leproult R, L'Hermite-Baleriaux M, Van Cauter E, Spiegel K. **Adverse effects of two nights of sleep restriction on the hypothalamic-pituitary-adrenal axis in healthy men**. *Journal of Clinical Endocrinology and Metabolism.* 99(8); Pp 2861-2868. 2014.

16. Hakkinen K, Pakarinen A, Alen M, Kauhanen H, Komi P. **Neuromuscular and hormonal adaptations in athletes to strength training in two years**. *Journal of Applied Physiology.* 65(6); Pp 2406-2412. 1988.

17. Hakkinen K, Pakarinen A, Alen M, Kauhanen H, Komi P. **Neuromuscular and hormonal responses in elite athletes to two successive strength training sessions in one day**. *European Journal of Applied Physiology and Occupational Physiology.* 57(2); Pp 133-139. 1988.

18. Hakkinen K, Pakarinen A, Alen M, Kauhanen H, Komi P. **Daily hormonal and neuromuscular responses to intensive strength training in 1 week**. *International Journal of Sports Medicine.* 9(6); Pp 422-428. 1988.

19. Hakkinen K, Pakarinen. **Acute hormonal responses to two different fatiguing heavy resistance protocols in male athletes**. *Journal of Applied Physiology.* 74(2); Pp 882-887. 1993.

20. Hartman M, Clarke B, Bembens D, Kilgore J, Bemben N. **Comparisons between twice-daily and once daily training sessions in male weightlifters**. *International Journal of Sports Physiology and Performance.* 2(2); Pp 159-169. 2007.

21. Hartmann H, Wirth K, Klusemann M. **Analysis of the load on the knee joint and vertebral column with changes in depth and weight load.** *Journal of Sports Medicine.* 43; Pp 993-1008. 2013.

22. Horne et al. **Health effects of intermittent fasting hormesis or harm? A systematic review.** *American Journal of Clinical Nutrition.* 102(2); Pp 464-470. 2015.
23. Hussin N, Shahar S, Teng N, Noah W, Das S. **Efficacy of fasting and calorie restriction (FCR) on mood and depression among ageing men.** *Journal of Nutrition, Health and Ageing.* 17(8); Pp 674-680. 2013.
24. Izquierdo M, Ibanez J, Hakkinen K, Kraemer W, Ruesta M, Gorostiaga E. **Maximal strength and power, muscle mass, endurance, and serum hormones in weightlifters and road cyclists.** *Journal of Sport Sciences.* 22(5); Pp 465-478. 2004.
25. Jung et al. **The hypoglycemic effects of hesperidin and naringin are partly mediated by hepatic glucose-regulating enzymes in C57BL/KsJ-db/db mice.** *Journal of Nutrition.* 134(10); Pp 2499-2503. 2004.
26. Kennedy D, Scholey A, Tildesley N, Perry E, Wesnes K. **Modulation of modd and cognitive performance following acute administration of Melissa officinalis (lemon balm).** *Pharmacol Biochem Behav.* 72(4); Pp 953- 964. 2002.
27. Kennedy D, Little W, Scholey A. **Attenuation of laboratory-induced stress in humans after acute administration of Melissa officinalis (Lemon Balm).** *Psychosomatic Medicine.* 66(4); Pp 607-613. 2004.
28. Khan et al. **Cinnamon Improves Glucose and Lipids of People With Type 2 Diabetes.** *Diabetes Care.* 26(12); Pp 3215-3218. 2003.
29. Killick R, Hoyos C, Melehan K, Dungan G, Poh J, Liu P, **Metabolic and hormonal effects of 'catch-up' sleep in men with chronic, repetitive, lifestyle-driven sleep restriction.** *Clinical Endocrinology.* 83(4); Pp 498-507. 2015.
30. Kirwan J, del Aguila L. **Insulin signaling, exercise and cellular integrity.** *Biochemical Society Transactions.* 31(6); Pp 1281-1285. 2003.
31. Kondo et al. **Vinegar intake reduces body weight, body fat mass, and serum triglyceride levels in obese Japanese subjects.** *Bioscience Biotechnology and Biochemistry.* 73(8); Pp 1837-1843.2009.
32. Kraemer W, Volek J, French D, Rubin M, Sharman M, Gomez A, Ratamess N, Newton R, Jemiolo B, Craig B, Hakkinen K. **The effects of L-carnitine L-tartrate supplementation on hormonal responses to resistance exercise and recovery.** *Journal of Strength and Conditioning Research.* 17(3); Pp 455-462. 2003.
33. Kraemer W, Spiering B, Volek J, Ratamess N, Sharman M, Rubin M, French D, Silvestre R, Hatfield D Van Heest J, Vingren J, Judelson D, Deschenes M, Maresh C. **Androgenic responses to resistance exercise: effects of feeding and L-carnitine.** *Medicine and Science in Sports and Exercise.* 38(7); Pp 1288-1296.2006.

34. Lavin D. et al. **Fasting induces an anti-inflammatory effect on the neuroimmune system which a high fat diet prevents.** *Obesity.* 19(8); Pp 1586-1594. 2011.

35. Leproult R, Van Cauter E. **Effect of 1 week of sleep restriction on testosterone levels in young healthy men.** *JAMA.* 305(21); Pp 2173-2174. 2011.

36. Maggio M, Ceda G, Lauretani F, Cattabiani C, et al. **Magnesium and anabolic hormones in older men.** *Int Journal of Androl.* 34(6); p 594-600. 2011.

37. Martin A, Normand S, Sothier M, Peyrat J, Louche-Pelissier C, Laville M. **Is advice for breakfast consumption justified? Results from a short-term dietary and metabolic experiment in young healthy men.** *British Journal of Nutrition.* 84(3); Pp 337-344. 2000.

38. Martin B, Mattson M, Maudsley S. **Caloric restriction and intermittent fasting: Two potential diets for successful brain aging.** *Ageing Res Rev.* 5(3); Pp 332-353. 2006.

39. Mazzetti S, Douglas M, Yocum A, Harber M. **Effect of explosive versus slow contractions and exercise intensity on energy expenditure.** *Medicine and Science in Sports and Exercise.* 39(8); Pp 1291-1301. 2007.

40. Nair P, Khawale P. **Role of therapeutic fasting in women's health: An overview.** *Journal of Mid-Life Health.* 7(2); Pp 61-64. 2016.

41. Nielson F, Johnson L, Zeng H. **Magnesium supplementation improves indicators of low magnesium status and inflammatory stress in adults older than 51 years with poor quality of sleep.** *Magnesium Research.* 23(3); Pp 158-168. 2010.

42. Pilz S, Frisch S, Koertke H, Kuhn J, Dreier J, Obermayer-Pietsch B, Wehr E, Zittermann A. **Effect of vitamin D supplementation on testosterone levels in men.** Horm Metab Res. 43(3); Pp 223-225. 2011.

43. Prasad A, Mantzoros C, Beck F, Hess J, Brewer G. **Zinc status and serum testosterone levels of healthy adults.** Nutrition.12(5): Pp 344-8. 1996.

44. Rayssiguier R, Libako P, Nowacki W, Rock E. **Magnesium deficiency and metabolic syndrome: Stress and inflammation may reflect calcium activation.** *Magnesium Research.* 23(2); Pp 73-80. 2010.

45. Reynolds A, Dorrian J, Liu P, Van Dogen H, Wittert G, Harmer L, Banks S. **Impact of five nights of sleep restriction on glucose metabolism, leptin and testosterone in young adult men.** *PLoS One.* 7(7); e41418. 2012.

46. Sakai K, Fukami Y, Yamagishi S, Kaida Y, Adachi T, Ando R, Manabe R, Otsuka A, Sugi K, Ueda S, Okuda S. **Evidence for a positive association between serum carnitine and free testosterone levels**

in uremic men with hemodialysis. *Rejuvenation Research.* 16(3); Pp 200-205. 2013.

47. Sethi J, Yadav M, Sood S, Dahiva K, Singh V. **Effect of tulsi (Ocimum Sanctum Linn) on sperm count and reproductive hormones in male albino rabbits.** *International Journal of Ayurvedic Research.* 1(4); Pp 208-210. 2010.

48. Sibille K, Bartsch F, Reddy D, Fillingim R, Keil A. **Increasing neuroplasticity to bolster chronic pain treatment: A role for intermittent fasting and glucose administration.** *Journal of Pain.* 17(3); Pp 275-281. 2016.

49. Skoldstam L, Larsson L, Lindstrom F. **Effect of fasting and lactovegetarian diet on Rheumatoid arthritis.** *Arthritis Rheu.* 31; Pp 585-592. 1988.

50. Sofer et al. **Greater weight loss and hormonal changes after 6 months diet with carbohydrates eaten mostly at dinner.** *Obesity (Silver Spring).* 19(10); Pp 2006-2014. 2011.

51. **Topo E, Soricelli A, D'Aneillo A, Ronsini S, D'Aniello G. The role and molecular mechanism of D-aspartic acid in the release and synthesis of LH and testosterone in humans and rats.** *Reprod Biol Endocrinol.* 7(120); Pp 1477-1478. 2009.

52. Traba J et al. **Fasting and refeeding differentially regulate NLRP3 inflammasome activation in human subjects.** *The Journal of Clinical Investigation.* 125(12); Pp 4592-4600. 2015.

53. Trumble B, Cummings D, O'Connor K, Holman, Smith E, Kaplan H, Gurvens M. **Age-independent increases in male salivary testosterone during horticultural activity among Tsimane forager-farmers.** *Evol Hum Behav.* 34(5). 2013.

54. Van Cauter E, Spiegel K, Tasali E, Leproult R. **Metabolic consequences of sleep and sleep loss.** *Sleep Med.* 9(1); Pp 23-28. 2008.

55. Van Middendorp H, Kox M, Pickkers P, Evers A. **The role of outcome expectancies for a training program consisting of meditation, breathing exercises, and cold exposure on the response to endotoxin administration: a proof-of-principle study.** *Clinical Rheumatology.* 35(4); Pp 1081-1085. 2016.

56. Vani K, Karakula M, Syed R, Alharrbi K. **Clinical relevance of vitamin C among lead-exposed infertile men.** *Genet Test Mol Biomarkers.* 16(9); Pp 1001-1006. 2012.

57. Wankhede S, Langade D, Joshi K, Sinha S, Bhattacharyya S. **Examining the effect of Withania somnifera supplementation on muscle strength and recovery: a randomized controlled trial.** *Journal of the International Society of Sports Nutrition.* 12(43). 2015.

58. Wehr E, Pilz S, Boehm B, Marz W, Obermayer-Pietsch B. **Association of vitamin D status with serum androgen levels in men.** *Clinical Endocrinology.* 73(2); Pp 243-248. 2010.

59. WD M, FI K, VL K. **Exercise Physiology: Energy, Nutrition, and Human Performance.** 7th ed. Baltimore, MD: *Lippincott Williams & Wilkins*; 2007.

60. Yun-Hee Youm et al. **Ketone body β-hydroxybutyrate blocks the NLRP3 inflammasome-mediated inflammatory disease.** *Natural Medicine.* 21(3); Pp 263–269. 2015.

Chapter 5 References

1. Garrido M, Espino J, Gonzalez-Gomez D, Lozano M, Barriga C, Paredes S, Rodriguez A. **The consumption of a Jerte Valley cherry product in humans enhances mood, and increases 5-hydroxyindoleacetic acid but reduces cortisol levels in urine.** *Experimental Gerontology.* 47(8); Pp 573-580. 2012

2. Hintzpeter J, Stapelfeld C, Loerz C, Martin H, Maser E. **Green tea and one of its constituents, Epigallocatechine-3-gallate, are potent inhibitors of human 11β-hydroxysteroid dehydrogenase type 1.** *PloS One.* 9(1); Pp e4468. 2014.

3. Jacka F, O'Neil A, Opie R, Itsiopoulos C, Cotton S, Mohebbi M, Castle D, Dash S, Mihalopoulos C, Chatterton M, Brazionis L, Dean O, Hodge A, Berk M. **A randomised controlled trial of dietary improvement for adults with major depression (the 'SMILES' trial).** *BMC Med.* 15(1); Pp 1-13. 2017.

4. Matsumura K, Yamakoshi T, Noguchi H, Rolfe P, Matsuoka Y. **Fish consumption and cardiovascular response during mental stress.** *BMC Research Notes.* 13(5);Pp 288. 2012.

5. Oi-Kano Y, Kawada T, Watanabe T, Koyama F, Watanabe K, Senbongi R, Iwai K. **Oleuropein supplementation increases urinary noradrenaline and testicular testosterone levels and decreases plasma corticosterone levels in rats fed high-protein diet.** *Journal of Nutritional Biochemistry.* 24(5); Pp 887-893. 2013.

6. Oi Y, Imafuku M, Shishido C, Kominato Y, Nishimura S, Iwai K. **Garlic supplementation increases testicular testosterone and decreases plasma corticostereone in rats fed a high protein diet.** *The Journal of Nutrition.* 131(8); Pp 2150-2156. 2001.

7. von Kanel R, Meister R, Arpagaus A, Treichler S, Kuebler U, Huber S, Ehlert U. **Dark chocolate intake buffers stress reactivity in humans.** *Journal of the American College of Cardiology.* 63(21); Pp 2297-2299. 2014.

40328173R00113

Made in the USA
Middletown, DE
25 March 2019